I0130181

Nursing Fundamentals Made Easy

Essential Skills for Nurses

Gina Renee Hawkins

© 2025 Gina Renee Hawkins. All rights reserved. No part of this publication may be reproduced, distributed, or transmitted in any form without written permission, except for brief quotations used in reviews and noncommercial purposes as permitted by law.

This book is for educational use only. It is not a substitute for formal nursing education, clinical training, or professional medical advice, diagnosis, or treatment. Readers should always consult qualified professionals, follow institutional protocols, and stay up-to-date with evolving standards.

Information is based on widely accepted practices at the time of publication, but healthcare changes rapidly. Users should verify all content using trusted sources, consult current guidelines, and prioritize patient safety. Clinical decisions must be based on professional judgment, current best practices, and institutional policies.

All case studies and examples are fictional and intended for teaching purposes only. Any similarities to real people, patients, or institutions are purely coincidental.

References to professionals (e.g., Florence Nightingale, Hildegard Peplau, Madeleine Leininger) are for educational context only and do not imply endorsement. Mention of organizations (e.g., ANA, NLN, CDC, WHO, The Joint Commission, NCSBN) is for informational purposes and does not suggest affiliation or approval.

All medication and treatment references are for general education. Verify drug details with updated resources, consult appropriate professionals, follow protocols, and consider allergies or contraindications.

Legal and regulatory details are general and vary by region. Nurses must comply with local laws, licensing regulations, and professional standards, and seek legal counsel when necessary.

The author and publisher are not responsible for any harm, loss, or injury resulting from the use of this book. Liability is disclaimed for all types of damages, including clinical errors or professional consequences.

Isohan Publishing

ISBN: 978-1-7642100-5-8

Table of Contents

Chapter 1: Introduction to Professional Nursing

The moment you step into a hospital, clinic, or any healthcare setting, you notice something special about the nurses. They move with purpose, speak with confidence, and somehow manage to be everywhere at once (or so it seems). But here's what you might not realize: every single one of these professionals started exactly where you are now—as a beginner wondering what nursing really means and how to become good at it.

Professional nursing isn't just about following orders or completing tasks. It's about understanding your role in healing, your responsibility to patients, and your commitment to a profession that shapes lives every single day. The American Nurses Association tells us that nursing is "the protection, promotion, and optimization of health and abilities, prevention of illness and injury, alleviation of suffering through the diagnosis and treatment of human response, and advocacy in the care of individuals, families, communities, and populations" (1). That's a mouthful, but it boils down to this: nurses help people feel better, get better, and stay better.

You're not just learning to be a helper—you're learning to be a professional. And there's a big difference between the two.

The Nursing Profession

Historical Evolution of Nursing

Picture this: It's 1860, and a determined woman named Florence Nightingale is walking through the dark corridors of a military hospital. She carries a lamp—not because she wants to look dramatic, but because she understands something other people don't. Light means cleanliness, organization, and hope. That lamp became the symbol of nursing, and it still guides us today.

But nursing didn't start with Florence Nightingale, and it certainly didn't stop with her. The profession has grown and changed in remarkable ways. In the early 1900s, nurses were primarily seen as assistants to physicians. They followed orders, kept patients comfortable, and rarely questioned medical decisions. By the 1950s, nurses like Hildegard Peplau began to challenge this model. She argued that nurses had their own unique knowledge and skills—that nursing was a science, not just a service.

The 1960s brought the civil rights movement, and nursing wasn't left behind. Nurses began demanding equal pay, better working conditions, and recognition of their expertise. The 1970s saw the rise of nurse practitioners—nurses who could diagnose and treat patients independently. The 1980s and 1990s brought evidence-based practice, which means nurses started using research to guide their care decisions.

Today, nursing is recognized as both an art and a science. We have our own theories, our own research, and our own ways of understanding health and illness. We're no longer just following orders—we're making clinical judgments, advocating for patients, and leading healthcare teams.

Here's what this means for you: When you become a nurse, you're joining a profession with a rich history of advocacy, innovation, and caring. You're not just learning skills—you're learning to think like a nurse.

Practical Exercise: Create a Timeline Poster of Nursing History

Take a large piece of paper and create a timeline starting from 1860 to today. Include these key events:

- 1860: Florence Nightingale establishes modern nursing principles
- 1909: First university-based nursing program at University of Minnesota
- 1952: Hildegard Peplau publishes "Interpersonal Relations in Nursing"

- 1965: First nurse practitioner program at University of Colorado
- 1999: Institute of Medicine report "To Err is Human" emphasizes patient safety
- 2010: Affordable Care Act increases demand for preventive care

Add pictures, quotes, or symbols for each era. This visual reminder will help you understand how nursing has evolved and where you fit in this ongoing story.

Contemporary Nursing Practice

Today's nursing practice looks very different from what it was fifty years ago. Modern nurses work in hospitals, clinics, schools, homes, and communities. They specialize in areas like critical care, pediatrics, mental health, and gerontology. Some nurses work directly with patients, while others focus on education, research, or administration.

The scope of nursing practice varies from state to state, but all nurses share certain responsibilities. According to the National Council of State Boards of Nursing, every nurse must be able to assess patients, plan care, implement interventions, and evaluate outcomes (2). This is called the nursing process, and it's the foundation of everything we do.

But here's what makes nursing unique: We don't just treat diseases— we care for people. We look at the whole person, not just their symptoms. We consider their fears, their family, their culture, and their goals. This is what we call holistic care, and it's what sets nursing apart from other healthcare professions.

State boards of nursing regulate our practice through licensing. When you graduate from nursing school, you'll take the NCLEX-RN exam to prove you're ready to practice safely. Once you pass, you'll receive a license that allows you to work in your state. Some states participate in the Nurse Licensure Compact, which means your license is valid in multiple states (3).

Case Study: Maria's Journey - From Nursing Student to Licensed RN

Meet Maria, a 23-year-old nursing student in her final semester. She's excited but nervous about becoming a "real nurse." During her clinical rotation in the cardiac unit, Maria cares for Mr. Johnson, a 65-year-old man recovering from heart surgery.

On her first day, Maria focuses on completing her assigned tasks: checking vital signs, giving medications, and documenting care. She's efficient but feels like she's just going through the motions. Her instructor, Ms. Chen, notices this and sits down with Maria.

"Tell me about Mr. Johnson," Ms. Chen says.

"He's post-op day two from cardiac surgery. His vital signs are stable, and he's tolerating clear liquids," Maria responds.

"What else do you know about him?"

Maria thinks for a moment. "Well, he seems worried about something. He keeps asking about his wife, and he hasn't been sleeping well."

"And what did you do about that?"

"I... I didn't do anything. I just documented it."

Ms. Chen smiles. "This is where nursing begins. You noticed something important—his emotional state. What could you do to help?"

Maria realizes she could sit with Mr. Johnson, listen to his concerns, and perhaps arrange for his wife to visit. She could also talk to the social worker about his worries. Over the next few days, Maria learns to see beyond the tasks to the person.

By the end of her rotation, Maria understands that nursing isn't just about completing assignments—it's about seeing the whole person and responding to their needs. She's learned to think like a nurse.

Three months later, Maria passes her NCLEX-RN exam and starts her first job on the same cardiac unit. She's still learning, but she knows she's not just a task-completer—she's a professional nurse.

This story illustrates how nursing education transforms students from task-oriented workers into professional nurses who can think critically and provide holistic care.

Professional Organizations

Nursing has numerous professional organizations that support, educate, and advocate for nurses. The American Nurses Association (ANA) is the largest and most influential. Founded in 1896, the ANA represents all registered nurses and works to advance the profession through policy, education, and advocacy (4).

The ANA has developed several important documents that guide nursing practice:

- The Code of Ethics for Nurses, which outlines our professional values and responsibilities
- The Standards of Practice, which describe what nurses should do
- The Standards of Professional Performance, which describe how nurses should behave

The National League for Nursing (NLN) focuses specifically on nursing education. They accredit nursing programs, develop educational standards, and provide resources for nursing faculty (5). If you're in nursing school, your program is likely accredited by either the NLN or the Commission on Collegiate Nursing Education (CCNE).

Specialty nursing organizations serve nurses in specific areas of practice. For example:

- The American Association of Critical-Care Nurses (AACN) serves nurses in intensive care units
- The Emergency Nurses Association (ENA) supports nurses in emergency departments
- The American Psychiatric Nurses Association (APNA) advocates for mental health nurses

These organizations provide continuing education, certification programs, and networking opportunities. They also advocate for policies that affect their specialty areas.

Activity: Research and Present on One Nursing Organization

Choose one nursing organization that interests you. Research their history, mission, and current activities. Prepare a five-minute presentation that answers these questions:

1. When was the organization founded and why?
2. What is their mission or purpose?
3. What services do they provide to members?
4. How do they advocate for the profession?
5. What opportunities do they offer for students?

Present your findings to your classmates. This exercise will help you understand the breadth of nursing organizations and may help you identify groups you'd like to join as a professional nurse.

Educational Standards and Competencies

NCLEX-RN Test Plan Framework

The National Council Licensure Examination for Registered Nurses (NCLEX-RN) is more than just a test—it's your gateway to professional practice. The exam is designed to determine if you have the knowledge, skills, and abilities to practice safely as a newly licensed nurse (6).

The NCLEX-RN is built around a framework that reflects real nursing practice. Instead of testing isolated facts, it evaluates your ability to make clinical judgments in realistic situations. The exam covers four major client needs categories:

Safe and Effective Care Environment (Management of Care and Safety and Infection Control) makes up about 20-30% of the exam. This includes questions about patient safety, infection control, legal and ethical issues, and coordinating care.

Health Promotion and Maintenance accounts for about 9-15% of the exam. These questions focus on growth and development, health screening, and disease prevention.

Psychosocial Integrity comprises about 9-15% of the exam. This area covers mental health concepts, coping mechanisms, and cultural considerations.

Physiological Integrity (Basic Care and Comfort, Pharmacological and Parenteral Therapies, Reduction of Risk Potential, and Physiological Adaptation) makes up about 50-62% of the exam. This is the largest category and includes questions about nutrition, medication administration, and managing illness.

The exam also integrates several processes throughout all categories:

- Clinical judgment and decision-making
- Caring and communication
- Teaching and learning
- Culture and spirituality

The NCLEX-RN uses a computerized adaptive testing format, which means the difficulty of questions adjusts based on your performance. If you answer a question correctly, the next question will be slightly more difficult. If you answer incorrectly, the next question will be easier. This continues until the computer determines with 95% confidence that you're either above or below the passing standard.

Assessment Tool: NCLEX-Style Practice Questions

Here's a sample question in NCLEX format:

A nurse is caring for a client who has been diagnosed with pneumonia. Which of the following actions should the nurse take first?

A) Administer prescribed antibiotic B) Encourage increased fluid intake C) Assess oxygen saturation D) Provide patient education about pneumonia

The correct answer is C) Assess oxygen saturation. This question tests your understanding of nursing priorities using the ABC framework (Airway, Breathing, Circulation). Before implementing any interventions, you must first assess the patient's condition.

Practice questions like this regularly to develop your test-taking skills and clinical judgment abilities.

QSEN Competencies Integration

The Quality and Safety Education for Nurses (QSEN) initiative was developed to prepare nurses for the 21st century healthcare environment. QSEN identifies six core competencies that every nurse should develop (7):

Patient-Centered Care means recognizing the patient as the source of control and full partner in providing compassionate and coordinated care. This involves understanding the patient's preferences, values, and needs.

Teamwork and Collaboration involves functioning effectively within nursing and interprofessional teams to foster open communication and shared decision-making.

Evidence-Based Practice means integrating best current evidence with clinical expertise and patient values to guide healthcare decisions.

Quality Improvement involves using data to monitor care outcomes and designing and implementing changes to continuously improve care.

Safety means minimizing risk of harm to patients through system effectiveness and individual performance.

Informatics involves using information and technology to communicate, manage knowledge, and support decision-making.

These competencies aren't separate skills—they work together in every aspect of nursing practice. For example, when you're giving a medication, you're using:

- Patient-centered care (considering the patient's preferences and concerns)
- Evidence-based practice (using research to guide your actions)
- Safety (following the rights of medication administration)
- Informatics (using technology to verify orders and document care)

Skill Building: QSEN Competency Self-Assessment Checklist

Rate yourself on each competency using this scale: 1 = Beginning level 2 = Developing level 3 = Proficient level 4 = Advanced level

Patient-Centered Care:

- I can assess patient preferences and values
- I can involve patients in care decisions
- I can advocate for patient needs
- I can provide culturally sensitive care

Teamwork and Collaboration:

- I can communicate effectively with team members
- I can participate in team meetings
- I can recognize my role within the team
- I can seek help when needed

Evidence-Based Practice:

- I can locate reliable sources of information
- I can evaluate the quality of evidence
- I can apply evidence to clinical decisions
- I can share evidence with others

Quality Improvement:

- I can identify opportunities for improvement
- I can participate in quality improvement activities
- I can use data to evaluate care
- I can implement changes to improve outcomes

Safety:

- I can identify potential safety hazards
- I can follow safety protocols
- I can communicate safety concerns
- I can participate in error reporting

Informatics:

- I can use electronic health records effectively
- I can access and evaluate online information
- I can use technology to support patient care
- I can protect patient privacy and confidentiality

Use this checklist at the beginning and end of each semester to track your progress. Don't worry if you're at the beginning level now—that's exactly where you should be as a student.

AACN Essentials Overview

The American Association of Colleges of Nursing (AACN) has developed The Essentials: Core Competencies for Professional Nursing Education, which provides a framework for nursing education at all levels (8). These essentials are organized into ten domains:

Domain 1: Knowledge for Nursing Practice involves understanding the scientific foundation of nursing, including pathophysiology, pharmacology, and health assessment.

Domain 2: Person-Centered Care focuses on providing care that is respectful, individualized, and based on patient preferences.

Domain 3: Population Health addresses the health of groups and communities, including health promotion and disease prevention.

Domain 4: Scholarship for Nursing Practice involves using evidence and research to improve nursing practice.

Domain 5: Quality and Safety emphasizes continuous improvement and risk reduction in healthcare.

Domain 6: Interprofessional Partnerships involves working collaboratively with other healthcare professionals.

Domain 7: Systems-Based Practice focuses on understanding how healthcare systems work and how to navigate them effectively.

Domain 8: Information and Healthcare Technologies involves using technology to support patient care and improve outcomes.

Domain 9: Professionalism encompasses the values, behaviors, and attitudes that characterize professional nurses.

Domain 10: Personal, Professional, and Leadership Development involves ongoing growth and development as a professional nurse.

These domains provide a roadmap for your nursing education. As you progress through your program, you'll develop competencies in each area. Don't expect to master everything at once—professional development is a lifelong process.

Progressive Element: Domain Tracking Throughout Program

Create a portfolio with ten sections, one for each domain. Throughout your nursing program, add evidence of your learning in each area. This might include:

- Reflection papers
- Care plans
- Research projects
- Clinical evaluations
- Certificates of completion

This portfolio will help you track your progress and prepare for job interviews after graduation.

Professional Identity Development

Values and Ethics

Nursing is more than a job—it's a calling that requires you to make ethical decisions every day. The ANA Code of Ethics for Nurses provides guidance for these decisions (9). The code includes nine provisions that address our responsibilities to patients, ourselves, and the profession.

Provision 1 states that nurses practice with compassion and respect for the inherent dignity, worth, and unique attributes of every person. This means treating all patients with kindness, regardless of their background, condition, or behavior.

Provision 2 requires that the nurse's primary commitment is to the patient. This means putting the patient's needs above your own convenience or preferences.

Provision 3 emphasizes that nurses must advocate for, and protect the rights of, patients. This includes protecting their privacy, ensuring informed consent, and speaking up when you see unsafe practices.

Provision 4 requires that nurses be responsible and accountable for their practice. This means admitting mistakes, staying current with best practices, and seeking help when needed.

Provision 5 states that nurses owe the same duties to themselves as to others. This includes maintaining your physical and mental health, continuing your education, and setting appropriate boundaries.

Provision 6 emphasizes that nurses must work to improve healthcare environments and conditions of employment. This might involve participating in quality improvement activities or advocating for better working conditions.

Provision 7 requires that nurses advance the profession through research, education, and practice development. This includes sharing your knowledge with students and colleagues.

Provision 8 states that nurses must collaborate with other health professionals to improve community, national, and international health. This emphasizes our role in addressing broader health issues.

Provision 9 emphasizes that the profession of nursing must articulate values, maintain integrity, and integrate principles of social justice into practice and policy. This includes addressing health disparities and advocating for vulnerable populations.

The MORAL framework provides a systematic approach to ethical decision-making (10):

- **M**assage the dilemma (identify the ethical problem)
- **O**utline the options (consider all possible actions)
- **R**esolve the dilemma (choose the best option)
- **A**ct by applying the chosen option
- **L**ook back and evaluate the results

Case Study: Boundary Dilemma - Gift from Grateful Patient

Sarah, a new nurse on the orthopedic unit, has been caring for Mrs. Martinez, an elderly woman recovering from hip replacement surgery.

Over the past week, Sarah has provided excellent care, and Mrs. Martinez has become quite fond of her. She often tells Sarah about her grandchildren and shares stories about her late husband.

On the day of discharge, Mrs. Martinez hands Sarah a small wrapped box. "This was my grandmother's ring," she says. "I want you to have it because you've been so kind to me. You remind me of my granddaughter."

Sarah is touched by the gesture but unsure about accepting the gift. She knows that patients sometimes offer gifts as a way to express gratitude, but she's not sure if accepting it would be appropriate.

Using the MORAL framework:

Massage the dilemma: The ethical issue is whether Sarah should accept a valuable personal gift from a patient. This involves questions about professional boundaries, patient autonomy, and the therapeutic relationship.

Outline the options:

1. Accept the gift graciously
2. Decline the gift and explain why
3. Accept the gift but donate it to charity
4. Consult with her supervisor before deciding

Resolve the dilemma: Sarah should decline the gift politely. While Mrs. Martinez's gesture is meaningful, accepting valuable gifts from patients can blur professional boundaries and create the appearance of favoritism.

Act by applying the chosen option: Sarah says, "Mrs. Martinez, I'm so touched that you want to give me something special. Your kind words mean more to me than any gift could. I think your granddaughter would love to have this beautiful ring."

Look back and evaluate: Mrs. Martinez understands and appreciates Sarah's professionalism. Their therapeutic relationship remains appropriate, and Sarah has maintained professional boundaries while still acknowledging the patient's gratitude.

This scenario illustrates how ethical principles guide nursing practice and help maintain appropriate relationships with patients.

Accountability and Responsibility

As a professional nurse, you'll be held accountable for your actions—both legally and ethically. This means you must practice within your scope of practice, follow established standards, and take responsibility for your decisions.

Legal implications in nursing include understanding your state's nurse practice act, which defines what nurses can and cannot do. You must also understand concepts like negligence, malpractice, and informed consent. Documentation is particularly important from a legal standpoint—if you don't document something, it's as if it never happened.

Documentation requirements vary by setting, but all healthcare organizations have policies about what must be documented and how. Good documentation is factual, timely, and complete. It should describe what you observed, what you did, and how the patient responded.

Delegation principles become important as you advance in your career. The National Council of State Boards of Nursing has developed five rights of delegation (11):

1. Right task (can be delegated safely)
2. Right circumstances (appropriate patient and setting)
3. Right person (qualified to perform the task)
4. Right direction (clear instructions given)
5. Right supervision (appropriate follow-up provided)

Remember: you can delegate tasks, but you can't delegate responsibility. You're still accountable for the outcomes.

Practical Exercise: Role-Play Delegation Scenarios

Work with a partner to practice delegation scenarios:

Scenario 1: You're a nurse on a medical unit with a certified nursing assistant (CNA). Mr. Johnson needs help with his bath, vital signs taken, and assistance walking to the bathroom. Which tasks can you delegate to the CNA?

Scenario 2: You're working in a busy emergency department. A patient needs an IV started, discharge teaching about medications, and a wound dressing changed. A nursing student is available to help. What can you delegate?

Scenario 3: You're the charge nurse on a surgical unit. You have two RNs and one LPN on your team. How would you divide the patient assignments?

Practice these scenarios until you feel comfortable making delegation decisions. Remember to consider the five rights of delegation in each situation.

Lifelong Learning

Nursing is a profession that requires continuous learning. Healthcare changes rapidly, and what you learn in nursing school is just the beginning. Most states require nurses to complete continuing education hours to maintain their licenses. But learning shouldn't stop there.

Continuing education requirements vary by state, but most require 20-30 hours of continuing education every two years. This can include formal courses, conferences, workshops, or online learning modules. Some states also require specific topics, such as domestic violence or pain management.

Professional development planning involves setting goals for your career and creating a plan to achieve them. This might include pursuing additional certifications, earning a higher degree, or developing expertise in a particular area.

Reflective practice is a key component of professional development. This involves thinking critically about your experiences, identifying areas for improvement, and developing strategies for growth. Many nurses keep journals or participate in peer review activities to support reflective practice.

Assessment Tool: Professional Development Portfolio Template

Create a portfolio with the following sections:

Section 1: Professional Goals

- Short-term goals (1-2 years)
- Long-term goals (5-10 years)
- Action steps for each goal

Section 2: Continuing Education Record

- Formal courses completed
- Conferences attended
- Certifications earned
- Online learning modules completed

Section 3: Professional Activities

- Committee memberships
- Volunteer activities
- Mentoring relationships
- Leadership roles

Section 4: Reflective Practice

- Critical incidents and lessons learned
- Peer feedback
- Self-assessments

- Personal growth observations

Section 5: Evidence of Competency

- Performance evaluations
- Letters of recommendation
- Awards or recognition
- Patient feedback

Update your portfolio regularly and use it to guide your professional development decisions.

Chapter 1 Skills Assessment

Your understanding of professional nursing concepts can be evaluated through several methods:

Competency Checklist: Professional Behavior Evaluation

Rate yourself on each behavior using this scale:

- Consistently demonstrates (3 points)
- Sometimes demonstrates (2 points)
- Rarely demonstrates (1 point)
- Never demonstrates (0 points)

Professional behaviors include:

- Arrives on time and prepared
- Dresses appropriately for the setting
- Communicates respectfully with patients and colleagues
- Maintains patient confidentiality
- Follows institutional policies and procedures
- Seeks help when needed
- Admits mistakes and learns from them
- Demonstrates cultural sensitivity
- Advocates for patient needs
- Participates in quality improvement activities

Critical Thinking Exercise: Ethical Dilemma Analysis

Read this scenario and apply the MORAL framework:

You're working the night shift in a medical unit. One of your patients, Mr. Thompson, is confused and keeps trying to get out of bed. His physician has ordered bed rest, but Mr. Thompson becomes agitated when restrained. His daughter, who is his healthcare proxy, insists that he be restrained "for his own safety." However, you know that restraints can increase confusion and risk of injury. What should you do?

Use the MORAL framework to analyze this situation and propose a solution.

Documentation Practice: Professional Goals Statement

Write a one-page professional goals statement that includes:

- Your vision of yourself as a professional nurse
- Your short-term and long-term career goals
- Your commitment to lifelong learning
- Your understanding of professional values and ethics

This statement should reflect your understanding of professional nursing and your commitment to the profession.

Key Takeaways

Professional nursing is built on a foundation of knowledge, skills, and values that have evolved over more than a century. As you begin your nursing journey, remember these essential points:

1. **Nursing is a profession, not just a job.** You're joining a community of professionals who are committed to improving health and alleviating suffering.

2. **Professional standards guide your practice.** The NCLEX-RN framework, QSEN competencies, and AACN essentials provide roadmaps for your development.
3. **Ethics are central to nursing practice.** The ANA Code of Ethics provides guidance for difficult decisions you'll face throughout your career.
4. **Accountability is personal.** You're responsible for your actions, your decisions, and your ongoing competence.
5. **Learning never stops.** Professional development is a lifelong commitment that begins in nursing school and continues throughout your career.

Understanding these concepts will help you develop a strong professional identity and provide safe, effective patient care. In the next chapter, we'll explore how healthcare systems work and how nurses collaborate with other professionals to provide comprehensive care.

Chapter 2: Healthcare Systems and Interprofessional Collaboration

Walk into any hospital at 7:00 AM and you'll witness something remarkable. Nurses gather in small groups, sharing information about patients who have been in their care all night. Physicians review charts and make rounds. Pharmacists verify medication orders. Therapists plan treatment sessions. Social workers coordinate discharge plans. And somehow, all of these different professionals work together to provide seamless care to patients.

This coordination doesn't happen by accident. It requires understanding how healthcare systems work, how different professionals contribute to patient care, and how to communicate effectively across disciplines. As a nurse, you'll be at the center of this complex web of relationships, often serving as the coordinator who ensures everyone is working toward the same goals.

Healthcare systems can seem overwhelming at first. There are different types of facilities, various payment methods, complex regulations, and constantly changing technologies. But once you understand the basics, you'll see that it's all designed around one central principle: providing the best possible care to patients and their families.

Healthcare Delivery Systems

Types of Healthcare Settings

Healthcare happens in many different places, each with its own unique characteristics and challenges. Understanding these settings will help you choose where you want to work and prepare you for the realities of different practice environments.

Acute care hospitals are what most people think of when they hear "hospital." These facilities provide 24-hour nursing care and medical services for patients with serious illnesses or injuries. They range from small community hospitals with 25 beds to large academic medical centers with over 1,000 beds. According to the American Hospital Association, there are approximately 6,090 hospitals in the United States (12).

In acute care settings, you'll see fast-paced environments where patient conditions can change rapidly. Nurses typically work 12-hour shifts and care for 4-6 patients, depending on the unit. The work is physically and emotionally demanding, but it's also rewarding because you can see the direct impact of your care on patient outcomes.

Long-term care facilities serve patients who need ongoing care but don't require the intensive services of a hospital. This includes nursing homes, skilled nursing facilities, and rehabilitation centers. About 1.3 million people live in nursing homes in the United States (13).

Long-term care nursing focuses on maintaining function, preventing complications, and supporting quality of life. You'll develop long-term relationships with residents and their families. The pace is generally slower than acute care, but the emotional challenges can be significant as you help people adjust to changes in their health and independence.

Community health centers provide primary care, preventive services, and health education to underserved populations. There are over 1,400 community health centers serving 30 million people nationwide (14). These centers often serve as a patient's primary entry point into the healthcare system.

Community health nursing emphasizes prevention, health promotion, and population health. You'll work with diverse populations and address social determinants of health like housing, food security, and education. The work is often focused on keeping people healthy rather than treating illness.

Home healthcare brings medical services directly to patients' homes. This rapidly growing field serves people who need skilled care but prefer to receive it at home rather than in a facility. The home healthcare industry employs over 3 million people and serves approximately 5 million patients annually (15).

Home health nursing requires independence and strong assessment skills because you're often the only healthcare provider in the home. You'll work with patients and families to manage chronic conditions, provide wound care, administer medications, and coordinate with other services.

Case Study: Mr. Thompson's Care Transition - Hospital to Home

Let's follow 78-year-old Mr. Thompson through his healthcare journey to understand how different settings work together.

Mr. Thompson lives alone in a small apartment. He has diabetes and heart disease, which are managed by his primary care physician at the local community health center. He visits the center every three months for check-ups and medication adjustments.

One evening, Mr. Thompson feels chest pain and shortness of breath. He calls 911 and is transported to the emergency department at Regional Medical Center, a 300-bed acute care hospital. The ED nurses quickly assess him and determine he's having a heart attack. He's taken to the cardiac catheterization lab, where a cardiologist opens a blocked artery and places a stent.

Mr. Thompson spends three days in the cardiac intensive care unit, where nurses monitor his heart rhythm, manage his medications, and help him understand what happened. On the fourth day, he's transferred to the medical unit, where nurses focus on education about his medications, diet, and activity restrictions.

The discharge planning team, which includes a nurse, social worker, and pharmacist, determines that Mr. Thompson needs additional support at home. They arrange for home health services to visit three times a week for the first month. The home health nurse will check his vital signs, review his medications, and assess his recovery progress.

After two weeks at home, Mr. Thompson returns to the community health center for follow-up care. His primary care physician reviews his hospital records, adjusts his medications, and refers him to a cardiac rehabilitation program at the local hospital.

This case illustrates how different healthcare settings work together to provide comprehensive care. Each setting has a unique role, but they all contribute to Mr. Thompson's recovery and long-term health.

Healthcare Team Members

Modern healthcare is delivered by teams of professionals, each with specialized knowledge and skills. Understanding these roles will help you collaborate effectively and advocate for your patients.

Physicians diagnose and treat medical conditions. They complete four years of medical school followed by residency training in their specialty. Primary care physicians include family medicine, internal medicine, and pediatrics doctors. Specialists focus on specific body systems or diseases.

Nurse practitioners are registered nurses with advanced education who can diagnose and treat patients independently in many states. They must complete a master's or doctoral degree in nursing and pass a national certification exam. There are over 290,000 nurse practitioners in the United States (16).

Physician assistants work under the supervision of physicians to provide diagnostic and therapeutic services. They complete a master's degree program and pass a national certification exam. There are approximately 131,000 physician assistants practicing in the United States (17).

Pharmacists are responsible for medication therapy management. They complete a Doctor of Pharmacy degree and are experts in drug interactions, side effects, and dosing. Clinical pharmacists work directly with healthcare teams to optimize medication therapy.

Physical therapists help patients recover movement and function after injury or illness. They complete a Doctor of Physical Therapy degree and focus on mobility, strength, and pain management.

Occupational therapists help patients regain the ability to perform activities of daily living. They complete a master's degree and focus on helping people adapt to disabilities or chronic conditions.

Social workers address psychosocial factors that affect health. They help patients navigate healthcare systems, access community resources, and cope with illness. Healthcare social workers typically have a master's degree in social work.

Respiratory therapists specialize in caring for patients with breathing problems. They operate ventilators, provide oxygen therapy, and perform breathing treatments.

Dietitians are nutrition experts who help patients manage diet-related health conditions. They complete a bachelor's degree in nutrition and complete an internship program.

Chaplains provide spiritual and emotional support to patients and families. They're trained in pastoral care and work with people of all faiths and belief systems.

Each team member brings unique expertise, but nurses often serve as the coordinators who ensure everyone is working together effectively. You'll spend the most time with patients, so you're often the first to notice changes in their condition or needs.

Practical Exercise: Interprofessional Team Simulation

Work in groups of 8-10 students, with each person taking on a different healthcare role. Use this scenario:

Mrs. Garcia, a 45-year-old woman with diabetes, is admitted to the hospital with a severe foot infection. She's been treated with antibiotics, but the infection isn't responding well. The physician is considering surgery, but Mrs. Garcia is afraid and wants to go home.

She speaks limited English and is worried about her three young children at home.

Each team member should contribute from their professional perspective:

- Physician: Medical diagnosis and treatment options
- Nurse: Patient assessment and care coordination
- Pharmacist: Antibiotic therapy recommendations
- Social worker: Childcare and language services
- Dietitian: Nutritional support for healing
- Physical therapist: Mobility and wound care
- Chaplain: Emotional and spiritual support

Discuss how each professional would contribute to Mrs. Garcia's care and how you would coordinate your efforts.

Patient Care Delivery Models

Healthcare organizations use different models to organize and deliver patient care. Understanding these models will help you adapt to different work environments and understand your role within the team.

Primary nursing assigns one nurse to be responsible for a patient's care throughout their hospital stay. This nurse assesses the patient, develops the care plan, and coordinates with other disciplines. When the primary nurse isn't working, an associate nurse provides care according to the established plan.

This model promotes continuity of care and allows nurses to develop therapeutic relationships with patients. However, it can be challenging to implement when nurses work different shifts or have varying levels of experience.

Team nursing divides patients among a team that includes registered nurses, licensed practical nurses, and nursing assistants. The team leader, usually an experienced RN, coordinates care and makes assignments based on patient needs and staff capabilities.

This model allows for efficient use of different skill levels and can be cost-effective. However, it requires strong leadership and communication skills to ensure coordinated care.

Case management assigns a nurse to coordinate care for specific patients throughout their entire healthcare episode, including hospital stay, discharge, and follow-up care. Case managers focus on ensuring patients receive appropriate care in the most cost-effective setting.

This model is particularly effective for patients with complex conditions or those at high risk for readmission. Case managers often work with patients across multiple settings and over extended periods.

Patient-centered medical homes organize primary care around comprehensive, coordinated, and accessible services. A primary care physician leads the team, but nurses play crucial roles in care coordination, patient education, and chronic disease management.

This model emphasizes prevention and proactive management of chronic conditions. Nurses often serve as care coordinators, helping patients navigate the healthcare system and manage their conditions at home.

Activity: Compare and Contrast Delivery Models

Create a chart comparing these four delivery models:

Model	Advantages	Disadvantages	Best Settings
Primary Nursing			
Team Nursing			
Case Management			
Patient-Centered Medical Home			

Consider factors like continuity of care, cost-effectiveness, patient satisfaction, and staff satisfaction. Discuss with your classmates which model you think would work best in different settings and why.

Communication in Healthcare

SBAR Communication Technique

Effective communication is essential for patient safety and quality care. The SBAR technique provides a structured framework for communicating important information clearly and concisely (18).

Situation: What is happening with the patient right now? **B**ackground: What is the relevant background information? **A**ssessment: What do I think the problem is? **R**ecommendation: What should we do to address the problem?

Let's break down each component:

Situation should include the patient's name, location, and a brief description of the current concern. Be specific and objective. For example: "This is Sarah calling about Mrs. Johnson in room 302. She's experiencing chest pain."

Background provides context for the current situation. Include relevant medical history, current medications, and recent changes in condition. For example: "Mrs. Johnson is a 65-year-old woman who had cardiac surgery two days ago. She was stable until about 30 minutes ago when she began complaining of chest pain."

Assessment includes your clinical findings and interpretation of the situation. Use objective data and avoid assumptions. For example: "Her vital signs are blood pressure 160/90, heart rate 110, respirations 24, and oxygen saturation 95% on room air. She appears anxious and is clutching her chest."

Recommendation should be specific and actionable. If you're not sure what to recommend, ask for specific guidance. For example: "I think she needs to be evaluated immediately. Should I give her nitroglycerin and call the physician, or would you like to see her first?"

The SBAR technique works because it mirrors the way healthcare providers think about clinical problems. It ensures that important information isn't missed and reduces the likelihood of miscommunication.

Skill Practice: SBAR Scenarios with Increasing Complexity

Practice using SBAR with these scenarios:

Scenario 1 (Simple): You're caring for Mr. Davis, who had knee replacement surgery yesterday. He's asking for pain medication, but he received his last dose two hours ago and isn't due for another dose for two hours.

Scenario 2 (Moderate): Mrs. Chen, who has diabetes, missed her breakfast and is now experiencing symptoms of low blood sugar. Her blood glucose is 65 mg/dL.

Scenario 3 (Complex): Mr. Rodriguez, who has a history of heart failure, is becoming increasingly short of breath. His oxygen saturation has dropped from 95% to 88%, and you notice swelling in his legs that wasn't there this morning.

Practice each scenario with a partner, with one person playing the nurse and the other playing the physician or charge nurse. Focus on providing clear, concise information that enables quick decision-making.

Assessment Tool: SBAR Competency Checklist

Use this checklist to evaluate SBAR communications:

Situation:

- States patient name and location
- Identifies self and role
- Describes current concern clearly
- Uses objective language

Background:

- Provides relevant medical history
- Includes current medications
- Describes recent changes
- Gives context for current situation

Assessment:

- Reports vital signs and objective findings
- Shares clinical observations
- Provides professional judgment
- Avoids assumptions

Recommendation:

- Makes specific suggestions
- Requests specific actions
- Asks clear questions
- Provides timeline for follow-up

Handoff Communication

Handoff communication occurs when responsibility for patient care is transferred from one healthcare provider to another. This might happen during shift changes, when patients are transferred between units, or when patients are discharged to another facility.

The **ISBARR** method expands on SBAR to include additional elements important for handoffs:

Introduction: Introduce yourself and your role Situation: Current patient condition Background: Relevant history and context Assessment: Your evaluation of the situation Recommendation:

Suggested actions or concerns **R**ead back: Confirm understanding of key points

Bedside shift report is becoming the standard practice in many hospitals. Instead of giving report in a separate room, nurses discuss patient care at the bedside, allowing the incoming nurse to see the patient and ask questions directly.

Benefits of bedside reporting include:

- Increased patient safety through better communication
- Improved patient satisfaction by involving them in their care
- Better continuity of care
- Opportunity for real-time problem-solving

Transfer communication occurs when patients move between departments or facilities. This requires comprehensive information about the patient's condition, treatment, and ongoing needs.

Practical Exercise: Mock Shift Change Reports

Work with a partner to practice shift change reports. Use this patient scenario:

Mr. Williams, 72 years old, room 215, admitted yesterday with pneumonia. He has a history of COPD and diabetes. He's receiving antibiotics and breathing treatments. His oxygen saturation has been stable at 94% on 2 liters of oxygen. He ate about 50% of his lunch and is concerned about his wife, who is in a nursing home. He's scheduled for a chest X-ray this afternoon.

Practice giving and receiving report, focusing on:

- Essential information for safe care
- Changes in patient condition
- Upcoming procedures or treatments
- Patient and family concerns
- Questions or concerns about the plan of care

Interprofessional Communication

Working with other healthcare professionals requires understanding their perspectives, respecting their expertise, and communicating in ways that promote collaboration.

Team huddles are brief meetings where team members share important information about patient care. These might occur at the beginning of each shift or whenever there's a significant change in patient status.

Effective huddles are:

- Brief (5-10 minutes)
- Focused on patient safety and quality
- Inclusive of all team members
- Action-oriented

Multidisciplinary rounds involve representatives from different disciplines meeting to discuss patient care plans. These rounds ensure that all perspectives are considered and that care is coordinated across disciplines.

Conflict resolution is sometimes necessary when team members disagree about patient care. Effective conflict resolution involves:

- Focusing on the patient's best interests
- Listening to all perspectives
- Seeking common ground
- Involving supervisors when necessary

Cultural considerations in team communication include understanding that different cultures may have different communication styles, decision-making processes, and attitudes toward authority.

Case Study: Language Barrier Team Challenge

The emergency department team is caring for Maria Santos, a 28-year-old woman who speaks only Spanish. She's experiencing abdominal pain, and the team suspects appendicitis. The physician wants to perform surgery, but Maria seems hesitant and keeps asking for her husband.

The team includes:

- Dr. Kim, the emergency physician
- Lisa, the emergency department nurse
- Carlos, the nursing assistant who speaks Spanish
- Sarah, the social worker

The team faces several challenges:

- Obtaining informed consent in Maria's primary language
- Understanding Maria's cultural beliefs about surgery
- Communicating with Maria's family
- Ensuring Maria understands the urgency of her condition

The team works together to address these challenges:

- A professional interpreter is called to ensure accurate communication
- The social worker contacts Maria's husband and helps him get to the hospital
- The team learns that Maria's culture emphasizes family involvement in medical decisions
- They adjust their approach to include Maria's husband in the decision-making process

This case illustrates how cultural differences can affect team communication and patient care. The team's willingness to adapt their approach led to better outcomes for Maria.

Systems-Based Practice

Quality and Safety Culture

Healthcare organizations are increasingly focused on creating cultures that prioritize patient safety and quality improvement. Understanding these concepts will help you contribute to positive change in your workplace.

Just culture principles recognize that most errors are caused by system problems rather than individual failures. This approach focuses on improving systems rather than blaming individuals, which encourages error reporting and learning (19).

Key elements of just culture include:

- Distinguishing between system failures and individual accountability
- Encouraging error reporting without fear of punishment
- Focusing on improvement rather than blame
- Supporting staff who are involved in adverse events

Error reporting systems allow healthcare workers to report safety concerns, near misses, and adverse events. These systems help organizations identify patterns and implement improvements.

Effective error reporting systems are:

- Non-punitive
- Confidential
- Easy to use
- Focused on system improvement

Root cause analysis is a systematic approach to understanding why adverse events occur. This process involves examining all factors that contributed to an event and developing action plans to prevent similar events.

Activity: Analyze a Sentinel Event Case

Review this case and identify contributing factors:

A patient received ten times the prescribed dose of insulin because the nurse misread a handwritten order. The patient experienced severe hypoglycemia and required emergency treatment.

Consider these factors:

- Individual factors (nurse's experience, fatigue, training)
- System factors (handwritten orders, medication storage, policies)
- Environmental factors (staffing, distractions, workload)
- Communication factors (order clarity, verification processes)

Develop recommendations to prevent similar events. Focus on system improvements rather than individual blame.

Healthcare Technology Systems

Technology plays an increasingly important role in healthcare delivery. Understanding these systems will help you provide safer, more efficient care.

Electronic health records (EHRs) store patient information electronically, making it accessible to all members of the healthcare team. EHRs can improve patient safety by providing alerts about drug interactions, allergies, and abnormal lab values.

Benefits of EHRs include:

- Improved legibility and accuracy of documentation
- Better coordination of care across providers
- Clinical decision support tools
- Easier access to patient information

Computerized provider order entry (CPOE) allows physicians to enter orders directly into the computer system. This reduces errors caused by illegible handwriting and provides immediate feedback about drug interactions or allergies.

Clinical decision support systems provide alerts and reminders to help healthcare providers make better decisions. These might include drug interaction warnings, allergy alerts, or reminders about preventive care.

Hands-on Practice: EHR Simulation Exercises

Practice using an EHR system with these activities:

1. **Patient lookup:** Find a patient's current medications, allergies, and recent lab results
2. **Documentation:** Record vital signs, assessment findings, and nursing interventions
3. **Order review:** Check new physician orders and identify any concerns
4. **Communication:** Send a secure message to another healthcare provider
5. **Reporting:** Generate a report about patient care activities

Focus on accuracy, efficiency, and understanding how the system supports patient safety.

Resource Management

Healthcare resources are limited, so it's important to use them wisely. This includes managing time, supplies, and human resources effectively.

Cost-effective care means providing the best possible outcomes while using resources efficiently. This doesn't mean cutting corners—it means avoiding waste and choosing interventions that provide the most benefit.

Supply management involves using supplies appropriately and avoiding waste. This includes:

- Using the right supplies for each procedure
- Checking expiration dates
- Avoiding unnecessary waste

- Reporting equipment problems promptly

Time management is crucial for providing safe, efficient care. Effective time management strategies include:

- Prioritizing tasks based on patient needs
- Clustering care activities to minimize interruptions
- Using technology to improve efficiency
- Delegating appropriate tasks to others

Progressive Element: Efficiency Tracking Throughout Clinical Experiences

Keep a log of your clinical experiences, noting:

- How you organized your patient care
- Time spent on different activities
- Strategies that worked well
- Areas for improvement
- Resource utilization

Review this log regularly with your instructor to identify patterns and develop more efficient approaches to patient care.

Chapter 2 Skills Assessment

Your understanding of healthcare systems and interprofessional collaboration can be evaluated through several methods:

OSCE Station: Interprofessional Communication Scenario

You'll be evaluated on your ability to communicate effectively with other healthcare professionals using this scenario:

You're the nurse caring for Mrs. Patterson, who is scheduled for surgery tomorrow. The surgeon has ordered her to stop eating and drinking after midnight, but she's diabetic and takes insulin. You're concerned about her blood sugar management overnight.

You need to:

- Use SBAR to communicate with the physician
- Involve the pharmacist in medication management
- Coordinate with the surgical team
- Document your communications

Documentation Practice: Team Communication Log

Keep a log of your communications with other healthcare professionals during your clinical experiences. Include:

- Date and time of communication
- Healthcare professional involved
- Method of communication (SBAR, phone, email, etc.)
- Issue or concern discussed
- Outcome or follow-up needed

Self-Assessment: Teamwork Effectiveness Scale

Rate yourself on these teamwork behaviors:

- Communicates clearly and respectfully
- Listens actively to others
- Asks for help when needed
- Offers help to teammates
- Shares information appropriately
- Respects others' expertise
- Participates in problem-solving
- Advocates for patients
- Maintains professional boundaries
- Contributes to a positive work environment

Key Takeaways

Understanding healthcare systems and interprofessional collaboration is essential for providing safe, effective patient care. Remember these important points:

1. **Healthcare delivery occurs in many settings,** each with unique characteristics and challenges. Understanding these settings will help you choose your career path and adapt to different environments.
2. **Effective communication is essential for patient safety.** Use structured communication techniques like SBAR to ensure important information is shared clearly and completely.
3. **Healthcare is delivered by teams of professionals,** each with specialized knowledge and skills. Respect others' expertise and understand your role within the team.
4. **Quality and safety culture requires everyone's participation.** Focus on system improvements rather than individual blame, and always prioritize patient safety.
5. **Technology supports but doesn't replace clinical judgment.** Use technology to enhance patient care while maintaining your critical thinking skills.
6. **Resource management is everyone's responsibility.** Use time, supplies, and human resources efficiently to provide cost-effective care.

Understanding these concepts will help you work effectively within healthcare systems and collaborate with other professionals to provide excellent patient care. In the next chapter, we'll explore how to conduct comprehensive health assessments—the foundation of all nursing care.

Chapter 3: Health Assessment Fundamentals

Imagin yourself walking into a patient's room for the first time. You have a stethoscope around your neck, a pen in your pocket, and a head full of nursing knowledge. But where do you start? How do you figure out what's really going on with this person? The answer lies in assessment—the cornerstone of all nursing care.

Health assessment isn't just about checking boxes on a form or gathering data for documentation. It's about understanding the whole person—their physical condition, their emotional state, their fears, their hopes, and their needs. Every intervention you'll ever perform, every decision you'll ever make, and every outcome you'll ever achieve starts with a thorough, thoughtful assessment.

The best nurses develop what we call "assessment eyes"—the ability to notice subtle changes, pick up on important cues, and see the bigger picture. This skill doesn't develop overnight, but with practice and patience, you'll learn to gather information systematically while building therapeutic relationships with your patients.

Assessment Foundations

Health History Components

The health history is like a story—your patient's story. It provides the context you need to understand their current health status and plan appropriate care. But gathering a health history requires more than just asking questions. It requires creating an environment where patients feel safe to share personal information.

Chief complaint and present illness form the opening chapter of your patient's story. The chief complaint is the reason the patient sought healthcare, usually described in their own words. For example, "I've been having chest pain for two hours" or "I can't catch my breath." The present illness expands on this complaint, exploring when it started, what makes it better or worse, and how it's affecting the patient's daily life.

Use the acronym **OLDCART** to explore symptoms systematically:

- **O**nset: When did it start?
- **L**ocation: Where is it?
- **D**uration: How long does it last?
- **C**haracter: What does it feel like?
- **A**ggravating factors: What makes it worse?
- **R**elieving factors: What makes it better?
- **T**iming: Does it follow a pattern?

Past medical history includes previous illnesses, surgeries, hospitalizations, and ongoing health conditions. This information helps you understand risk factors and potential complications. Don't just collect diagnoses—understand how these conditions affect the patient's current health.

Family history reveals genetic predispositions and inherited conditions. Focus on immediate family members and conditions that might be relevant to the patient's current health. For example, if your patient has chest pain, a family history of heart disease is particularly important.

Social history explores lifestyle factors that affect health, including occupation, living situation, support systems, and health habits. This information helps you understand the patient's resources and potential barriers to care.

Review of systems is a systematic assessment of each body system to identify symptoms the patient might not have mentioned. This comprehensive approach ensures you don't miss important information.

Practical Exercise: Structured Interview Practice with Peers

Work with a classmate to practice health history interviews. One person plays the patient, the other the nurse. Use this scenario:

The "patient" is a 45-year-old office worker who comes to the clinic complaining of frequent headaches that started about three weeks

41

ago. The headaches are worse in the morning and seem to be getting more frequent.

The "nurse" should:

- Create a comfortable environment for the interview
- Use open-ended questions to encourage discussion
- Follow up with specific questions using OLDCART
- Show empathy and active listening
- Gather information about past medical history and family history
- Explore social factors that might be relevant

Switch roles and practice with different scenarios. Focus on developing your interviewing skills and building rapport with patients.

Cultural Assessment

Healthcare happens within the context of culture, and effective assessment requires understanding how cultural factors influence health beliefs, behaviors, and communication styles. Cultural assessment isn't about stereotyping—it's about understanding each patient as an individual within their cultural context.

Cultural assessment models provide frameworks for understanding how culture affects health. Madeleine Leininger's Sunrise Model explores cultural and social factors that influence care, while the ETHNIC framework provides a systematic approach to cultural assessment (20):

- **E**xplanation: How does the patient explain their illness?
- **T**reatment: What treatments has the patient tried?
- **H**ealers: Who else has the patient consulted?
- **N**egotiate: How can you incorporate cultural preferences?
- **I**ntervention: What interventions respect cultural values?
- **C**ollaborate: How can you work with cultural healers?

42

Health beliefs and practices vary widely across cultures. Some cultures view illness as a natural part of life, while others see it as a spiritual problem. Some emphasize individual responsibility for health, while others focus on family or community involvement. Understanding these beliefs helps you provide culturally sensitive care.

Use of interpreters is essential when language barriers exist. Professional interpreters are trained to provide accurate, confidential translation without adding their own interpretations. They can also help you understand cultural nuances that might affect care.

Guidelines for working with interpreters include:

- Speak directly to the patient, not the interpreter
- Use first-person language ("How are you feeling?" not "How is she feeling?")
- Pause frequently to allow for translation
- Watch for non-verbal cues from the patient
- Confirm understanding through the interpreter

Case Study: Mrs. Rosas - Culturally Sensitive Cardiac Care

Mrs. Carmen Rosas, a 58-year-old Mexican-American woman, is admitted to the cardiac unit with chest pain. She's accompanied by her large extended family, including her husband, three adult children, and several grandchildren. The family seems very concerned and wants to stay with her constantly.

During the assessment, Mrs. Rosas speaks mainly Spanish, though she understands some English. She keeps looking to her husband before answering questions, and he sometimes answers for her. She seems reluctant to discuss her symptoms in detail and keeps saying "It's God's will."

The nursing assessment reveals several cultural factors that affect Mrs. Rosas's care:

Family involvement: In Mexican culture, family plays a central role in healthcare decisions. Mrs. Rosas's family isn't just visiting—they're participating in her care. Rather than seeing this as interference, the nurse recognizes it as a source of support.

Gender roles: Mrs. Rosas may be accustomed to her husband making decisions or speaking for her in public settings. The nurse respects this while also ensuring Mrs. Rosas has opportunities to express her own concerns.

Religious beliefs: Mrs. Rosas's references to "God's will" reflect her spiritual beliefs about illness and healing. The nurse doesn't dismiss these beliefs but explores how they might affect her willingness to participate in treatment.

Language preferences: While Mrs. Rosas understands some English, she's more comfortable expressing complex thoughts in Spanish. The nurse arranges for a professional interpreter to ensure accurate communication.

Pain expression: Some cultures discourage expressing pain or discomfort, which might affect Mrs. Rosas's willingness to report symptoms. The nurse uses multiple approaches to assess her pain level, including observation and family input.

The nurse adapts the assessment approach to respect Mrs. Rosas's cultural values while ensuring comprehensive care:

- Includes family members in discussions when appropriate
- Uses a professional interpreter for complex conversations
- Respects Mrs. Rosas's religious beliefs while providing medical information
- Allows time for family consultation before making decisions
- Incorporates cultural healing practices when possible

This culturally sensitive approach leads to better communication, increased trust, and more effective care for Mrs. Rosas.

Therapeutic Communication

Assessment isn't just about gathering information—it's about building relationships. Therapeutic communication techniques help you connect with patients, understand their concerns, and establish trust.

Active listening means giving your full attention to the patient. This involves:

- Maintaining appropriate eye contact
- Using open body language
- Avoiding interruptions
- Reflecting back what you hear
- Asking clarifying questions

Open-ended questioning encourages patients to share information in their own words. Instead of asking "Are you having pain?" try "Tell me about any discomfort you're experiencing." This approach often reveals information that closed-ended questions might miss.

Nonverbal communication includes facial expressions, body language, and tone of voice. Research shows that up to 93% of communication is nonverbal, so pay attention to both your nonverbal messages and your patient's (21).

Motivational interviewing basics help patients explore their own motivations for change. This approach is particularly useful when discussing lifestyle modifications or treatment compliance. Key principles include:

- Expressing empathy
- Developing discrepancy between current behavior and goals
- Rolling with resistance rather than confronting it
- Supporting self-efficacy

Skill Practice: Video-Recorded Patient Interviews with Feedback

Practice your communication skills by recording (with permission) practice interviews with standardized patients or classmates. Review the recordings to identify:

- Effective communication techniques
- Areas for improvement
- Nonverbal communication patterns
- Missed opportunities for therapeutic communication

Common areas for improvement include:

- Talking too much instead of listening
- Asking multiple questions at once
- Missing emotional cues
- Using medical jargon
- Appearing rushed or distracted

Physical Assessment Techniques

Inspection Skills

Inspection is the most basic but most important assessment technique. It involves using your senses—primarily sight, but also hearing and smell—to gather information about the patient.

Systematic observation means looking at the patient in an organized way. Start with general observations about the patient's overall appearance, then move to specific body systems. Notice:

- General appearance and behavior
- Skin color and condition
- Breathing patterns
- Posture and movement
- Facial expressions
- Hygiene and grooming

Normal vs. abnormal findings require knowledge of what's expected for different populations. Normal findings vary by age, gender, ethnicity, and individual variation. Abnormal findings might indicate disease, injury, or other health problems.

Documentation of observations should be objective, specific, and complete. Avoid subjective interpretations. For example, write "Patient grimaces when moving right arm" rather than "Patient appears to be in pain."

Assessment Tool: Body Systems Inspection Checklist

Use this systematic approach for inspection:

General Appearance:

- Level of consciousness and orientation
- Apparent age compared to stated age
- Nutritional status
- Posture and gait
- Dress and grooming

Skin:

- Color (pallor, cyanosis, jaundice, flushing)
- Moisture (dry, moist, diaphoretic)
- Temperature (warm, cool, hot)
- Texture (smooth, rough, thick, thin)
- Turgor (elastic, tented)
- Lesions or injuries

Head and Neck:

- Symmetry and proportion
- Hair distribution and texture
- Eye appearance and movement
- Facial expressions
- Neck position and movement

Chest:

- Shape and symmetry
- Breathing patterns
- Use of accessory muscles

- Skin color and condition

Extremities:

- Symmetry and proportion
- Muscle tone and strength
- Range of motion
- Swelling or deformity
- Skin condition

Practice this systematic approach until it becomes automatic. Consistent inspection helps you notice subtle changes that might indicate problems.

Palpation Techniques

Palpation uses touch to assess temperature, moisture, texture, size, shape, and movement. It's a skill that improves with practice and requires sensitivity and confidence.

Light palpation uses gentle pressure with the fingertips to assess surface characteristics. Use this technique to:

- Assess skin temperature and moisture
- Detect surface masses or swelling
- Evaluate muscle tone
- Check for tenderness

Deep palpation applies more pressure to assess deeper structures. Use this technique to:

- Evaluate organ size and shape
- Detect deep masses
- Assess muscle strength
- Check for deep tenderness

Assessing pulses requires understanding pulse locations and characteristics. Major pulse points include:

- Temporal (temple area)
- Carotid (neck)
- Brachial (inside upper arm)
- Radial (wrist)
- Femoral (groin)
- Popliteal (behind knee)
- Posterior tibial (inside ankle)
- Dorsalis pedis (top of foot)

Assess pulse rate, rhythm, and quality. Document findings using a standard scale:

- 0 = Absent
- 1+ = Weak/thready
- 2+ = Normal
- 3+ = Bounding

Lymph node examination involves palpating major lymph node groups to detect enlargement, tenderness, or other abnormalities. Major lymph node areas include:

- Head and neck
- Axillary (armpit)
- Epitrochlear (elbow)
- Inguinal (groin)

Hands-on Practice: Palpation Stations with Simulation Mannequins

Set up practice stations with different palpation scenarios:

Station 1: Pulse Assessment

- Practice finding all major pulse points
- Assess rate, rhythm, and quality
- Compare pulses bilaterally
- Document findings accurately

Station 2: Abdominal Palpation

49

- Practice light and deep palpation techniques
- Identify normal abdominal structures
- Detect abnormal masses or tenderness
- Assess for organomegaly

Station 3: Lymph Node Assessment

- Locate major lymph node groups
- Use proper palpation technique
- Identify normal vs. abnormal findings
- Document size, mobility, and tenderness

Station 4: Extremity Assessment

- Assess for edema using proper technique
- Evaluate muscle tone and strength
- Check for deformities or swelling
- Compare findings bilaterally

Practice these techniques regularly to develop confidence and skill. Remember that palpation can be uncomfortable for patients, so explain what you're doing and ask for permission before touching.

Percussion and Auscultation

Percussion and auscultation are advanced assessment techniques that require practice to master. These skills help you assess internal structures and functions.

Percussion techniques involve tapping on the body surface to produce sounds that reveal information about underlying structures. The technique uses a plexor finger (usually the middle finger) to strike a pleximeter finger (usually the middle finger of the other hand) placed on the patient's skin.

Percussion sounds vary depending on the density of underlying tissue:

- **Tympany:** High-pitched, drum-like sound over air-filled structures (stomach)
- **Resonance:** Low-pitched, hollow sound over normal lung tissue
- **Dullness:** Medium-pitched, thud-like sound over fluid or solid tissue (liver)
- **Flatness:** High-pitched, flat sound over very dense tissue (muscle)

Stethoscope use and care requires understanding different parts and their functions:

- **Diaphragm:** Detects high-pitched sounds (breath sounds, heart sounds)
- **Bell:** Detects low-pitched sounds (heart murmurs, bowel sounds)
- **Earpieces:** Should fit snugly and be angled toward your ear canals
- **Tubing:** Should be about 12 inches long and free of cracks

Heart sounds include:

- **S1:** "Lub" sound caused by closure of mitral and tricuspid valves
- **S2:** "Dub" sound caused by closure of aortic and pulmonary valves
- **S3:** Gallop rhythm that may indicate heart failure
- **S4:** Gallop rhythm that may indicate hypertension

Lung sounds include:

- **Vesicular:** Normal breath sounds over healthy lung tissue
- **Bronchial:** Normal breath sounds over large airways
- **Adventitious:** Abnormal sounds including crackles, wheezes, and rhonchi

Bowel sounds are gurgling sounds produced by intestinal movement. Normal bowel sounds occur every 5-15 seconds. Absent bowel sounds may indicate obstruction, while hyperactive sounds may indicate infection or obstruction.

Progressive Skill Building: Basic to Advanced Sound Identification

Start with basic sound identification and progress to more complex assessments:

Level 1: Basic Sounds

- Identify normal heart sounds (S1, S2)
- Recognize normal breath sounds
- Detect presence or absence of bowel sounds

Level 2: Intermediate Sounds

- Distinguish between different breath sound abnormalities
- Identify heart murmurs
- Assess bowel sound frequency and quality

Level 3: Advanced Sounds

- Differentiate between types of crackles
- Identify specific heart sound abnormalities
- Correlate sound findings with clinical conditions

Use audio recordings, simulation mannequins, and supervised practice with real patients to develop these skills progressively.

Vital Signs Mastery

Temperature Assessment

Body temperature reflects the balance between heat production and heat loss. Understanding normal variations and accurate measurement techniques is essential for patient assessment.

Methods and normal ranges vary depending on the measurement site:

- **Oral:** 98.6°F (37°C), range 97.0-99.5°F (36.1-37.5°C)
- **Rectal:** 99.6°F (37.6°C), range 98.0-100.4°F (36.7-38.0°C)
- **Axillary:** 97.6°F (36.4°C), range 96.0-98.4°F (35.6-36.9°C)
- **Tympanic:** 98.6°F (37°C), range 97.0-99.5°F (36.1-37.5°C)
- **Temporal:** 99.0°F (37.2°C), range 97.5-100.4°F (36.4-38.0°C)

Factors affecting temperature include:

- Time of day (lowest in early morning, highest in late afternoon)
- Age (infants and elderly have less stable temperatures)
- Gender (women have cyclical variations)
- Activity level (exercise increases temperature)
- Environmental conditions
- Illness or infection

Fever patterns provide diagnostic clues:

- **Intermittent:** Temperature returns to normal between fever episodes
- **Remittent:** Temperature varies but doesn't return to normal
- **Relapsing:** Fever episodes separated by normal temperature periods
- **Constant:** Temperature remains elevated with minimal variation

Practical Exercise: Temperature Measurement Relay

Set up stations with different thermometry methods:

Station 1: Oral Temperature

- Practice proper thermometer placement
- Ensure patient hasn't eaten, drunk, or smoked recently
- Wait appropriate time for accurate reading

- Document findings correctly

Station 2: Tympanic Temperature

- Practice proper ear pull technique (up and back for adults, down and back for children)
- Insert thermometer correctly
- Obtain accurate reading
- Clean equipment between uses

Station 3: Temporal Temperature

- Practice proper scanning technique
- Understand when to use behind-the-ear correction
- Recognize factors that affect accuracy
- Document findings appropriately

Station 4: Axillary Temperature

- Position thermometer correctly
- Ensure proper contact with skin
- Wait appropriate time for reading
- Understand limitations of this method

Rotate through stations to practice different techniques and understand when each method is most appropriate.

Pulse and Respiration

Pulse and respiration assessment provides information about cardiovascular and respiratory function. These vital signs are often assessed together because they're related and can be obtained simultaneously.

Pulse sites and characteristics include multiple locations where arterial pulsations can be felt. The radial pulse is most commonly used for routine assessment, but other sites may be necessary in specific situations.

Pulse characteristics to assess include:

- **Rate:** Normal adult rate is 60-100 beats per minute
- **Rhythm:** Should be regular with consistent intervals
- **Quality:** Should be strong and easily palpable

Respiratory patterns to observe include:

- **Eupnea:** Normal breathing pattern
- **Tachypnea:** Rapid breathing (>24 breaths per minute)
- **Bradypnea:** Slow breathing (<10 breaths per minute)
- **Apnea:** Absence of breathing
- **Dyspnea:** Difficult or labored breathing

Pulse oximetry principles involve measuring oxygen saturation of hemoglobin using light absorption. Normal oxygen saturation is 95-100% in healthy adults. Factors affecting accuracy include:

- Nail polish or artificial nails
- Poor circulation
- Motion artifacts
- Ambient light
- Carbon monoxide poisoning

Case Study: Identifying Respiratory Distress in Pediatric Patient

Eight-year-old Michael is brought to the emergency department by his parents. He's been having difficulty breathing for the past hour, and his parents are very worried. The triage nurse quickly assesses Michael's condition.

Initial observations:

- Michael is sitting upright, leaning forward
- He's using accessory muscles to breathe
- His breathing is rapid and shallow
- He appears anxious and restless
- His lips have a bluish tint

Vital signs:

- Heart rate: 140 beats per minute (normal for age: 70-110)
- Respiratory rate: 40 breaths per minute (normal for age: 16-20)
- Oxygen saturation: 88% on room air (normal: 95-100%)
- Temperature: 101.2°F (38.4°C)

Assessment findings: The nurse recognizes signs of respiratory distress:

- **Tachypnea:** Rapid breathing rate
- **Tachycardia:** Rapid heart rate (compensatory response)
- **Accessory muscle use:** Indicates increased work of breathing
- **Cyanosis:** Blue tint around lips indicates poor oxygenation
- **Positioning:** Sitting upright to ease breathing

Immediate interventions:

- Apply oxygen via nasal cannula
- Notify physician immediately
- Prepare for possible nebulizer treatment
- Position for comfort
- Reassure child and parents
- Continuously monitor vital signs

Follow-up: After receiving oxygen and bronchodilator treatment, Michael's condition improves:

- Respiratory rate decreases to 24 breaths per minute
- Oxygen saturation increases to 96%
- Accessory muscle use decreases
- Cyanosis resolves
- Child appears less anxious

This case demonstrates how vital signs assessment can quickly identify serious conditions and guide immediate interventions.

Blood Pressure Measurement

Blood pressure reflects the force of blood against arterial walls and provides important information about cardiovascular function. Accurate measurement requires proper technique and understanding of factors that affect readings.

Manual and automatic techniques both have advantages and limitations:

Manual measurement using a sphygmomanometer and stethoscope:

- Allows assessment of Korotkoff sounds
- More accurate in patients with irregular rhythms
- Requires skill and practice
- Time-consuming

Automatic measurement using electronic devices:

- Quick and convenient
- Reduces human error
- May be inaccurate in certain conditions
- Doesn't provide information about sound quality

Proper cuff sizing is critical for accurate readings:

- Cuff width should be 40% of arm circumference
- Cuff length should encircle 80% of arm circumference
- Wrong cuff size can cause significant errors in readings

Orthostatic vital signs assess for postural hypotension by measuring blood pressure and heart rate in lying, sitting, and standing positions. Significant changes may indicate:

- Dehydration
- Medication effects
- Autonomic dysfunction
- Blood loss

Common errors and troubleshooting include:

- Incorrect cuff size
- Improper cuff placement
- Rapid deflation
- Patient movement or talking
- Environmental noise
- Equipment malfunction

Skill Station: BP Measurement Competency with Various Patient Sizes

Practice blood pressure measurement with different scenarios:

Station 1: Adult Standard Size

- Practice proper cuff selection
- Position patient correctly
- Use proper technique for inflation and deflation
- Identify first and last Korotkoff sounds
- Document findings accurately

Station 2: Pediatric Patient

- Select appropriate cuff size
- Modify technique for child's comfort
- Recognize normal values for age
- Handle patient anxiety appropriately

Station 3: Obese Patient

- Choose correct cuff size
- Position cuff properly on large arm
- Use thigh cuff if necessary
- Recognize potential accuracy issues

Station 4: Patient with Irregular Rhythm

- Use manual technique when automatic fails
- Take multiple readings
- Identify irregular patterns

- Document findings appropriately

Station 5: Orthostatic Assessment

- Measure in all three positions
- Allow adequate time between positions
- Recognize significant changes
- Ensure patient safety during assessment

Pain Assessment

Pain is often called the "fifth vital sign" because it's so important to patient comfort and recovery. Effective pain assessment requires understanding different types of pain and using appropriate assessment tools.

Pain scales for different populations include:

- **Numeric Rating Scale (0-10):** Most common for adults
- **Visual Analog Scale:** Line marked from "no pain" to "worst possible pain"
- **Faces Pain Scale:** Pictures of faces showing different pain levels
- **FLACC Scale:** Observational tool for infants and nonverbal patients

PQRST method provides systematic pain assessment:

- Provocation/Palliation: What causes or relieves the pain?
- Quality: What does the pain feel like?
- Region/Radiation: Where is the pain? Does it spread?
- Severity: How intense is the pain on a scale of 0-10?
- Timing: When does the pain occur? How long does it last?

Cultural considerations in pain expression include:

- Some cultures encourage stoic responses to pain
- Others may express pain more dramatically
- Religious or spiritual beliefs may affect pain perception

- Gender roles may influence pain expression
- Previous experiences with healthcare may affect reporting

Activity: Create Age-Appropriate Pain Assessment Tools

Design pain assessment tools for different populations:

Tool 1: Preschool Children (3-5 years)

- Use simple language and concepts
- Include visual aids (faces, colors)
- Keep assessment brief
- Involve parents in assessment

Tool 2: School-Age Children (6-12 years)

- Use numeric scales with visual aids
- Explain the assessment process
- Allow child to participate actively
- Consider developmental level

Tool 3: Adolescents (13-18 years)

- Use adult-style numeric scales
- Respect privacy and independence
- Address concerns about addiction
- Consider peer influence

Tool 4: Older Adults

- Account for cognitive changes
- Use large, clear visual aids
- Allow extra time for response
- Consider multiple chronic conditions

Tool 5: Patients with Cognitive Impairment

- Use observational tools

- Look for behavioral indicators
- Involve family members
- Consider baseline behavior patterns

Documentation of Assessment

SOAP Documentation

SOAP (Subjective, Objective, Assessment, Plan) documentation provides a systematic approach to recording patient information. This format helps ensure comprehensive documentation and facilitates communication among healthcare providers.

Subjective data includes information the patient tells you:

- Chief complaint in patient's own words
- Symptoms described by patient
- Patient's perception of their condition
- Relevant history provided by patient
- Concerns expressed by patient or family

Objective data includes information you observe or measure:

- Vital signs and physical assessment findings
- Laboratory and diagnostic test results
- Observations about patient behavior
- Measurable outcomes
- Visual observations

Assessment includes your professional judgment about the patient's condition:

- Nursing diagnoses
- Analysis of subjective and objective data
- Identification of patient problems
- Evaluation of patient responses
- Clinical impressions

Plan includes interventions and expected outcomes:

- Specific nursing interventions
- Goals and expected outcomes
- Patient education plans
- Discharge planning considerations
- Follow-up requirements

Documentation Practice: Write SOAP Notes from Video Scenarios

Practice SOAP documentation using standardized scenarios:

Scenario 1: Post-operative patient with pain

- **S:** Patient states "I'm having severe pain in my incision, about 8 out of 10"
- **O:** Vital signs stable, grimacing with movement, guarding incision site
- **A:** Acute post-operative pain related to surgical incision
- **P:** Administer prescribed pain medication, reassess in 30 minutes, teach splinting techniques

Scenario 2: Patient with shortness of breath

- **S:** Patient reports "I can't catch my breath, especially when I walk"
- **O:** Respiratory rate 28, oxygen saturation 89%, crackles in lung bases
- **A:** Impaired gas exchange related to fluid overload
- **P:** Apply oxygen, elevate head of bed, notify physician, monitor respiratory status

Practice writing complete SOAP notes for various scenarios to develop documentation skills.

Electronic Documentation

Electronic health records (EHRs) have transformed healthcare documentation, offering advantages like improved legibility, clinical decision support, and better coordination of care. However, they also present challenges that nurses must understand.

EHR assessment templates standardize documentation and ensure comprehensive assessment. These templates typically include:

- Pre-populated normal findings
- Drop-down menus for common assessments
- Required fields for essential information
- Integration with other hospital systems
- Alerts for abnormal values

Avoiding copy-paste errors is crucial for patient safety:

- Always verify copied information is current and accurate
- Update assessment findings with each encounter
- Don't copy forward outdated information
- Customize templates for individual patients
- Review entries before finalizing

Hands-on Practice: Document Assessments in Simulated EHR

Practice using EHR systems with these activities:

Activity 1: Initial Assessment Documentation

- Navigate to assessment module
- Complete head-to-toe assessment documentation
- Use appropriate terminology and abbreviations
- Include all required elements
- Save and review documentation

Activity 2: Progress Note Documentation

- Document changes in patient condition
- Update assessment findings
- Record interventions and patient responses

- Use appropriate time stamps
- Ensure accuracy and completeness

Activity 3: Discharge Documentation

- Complete discharge assessment
- Document patient education provided
- Record discharge instructions
- Update care plan
- Ensure continuity of care information

Activity 4: Error Correction

- Practice making corrections using proper procedures
- Understand legal requirements for changes
- Document rationale for corrections
- Maintain audit trail
- Follow institutional policies

Chapter 3 Skills Assessment

Your competency in health assessment can be evaluated through multiple methods:

Comprehensive Health Assessment OSCE

You'll be evaluated on your ability to:

- Conduct a systematic health history interview
- Perform a complete physical assessment
- Document findings accurately
- Identify normal and abnormal findings
- Communicate effectively with patients
- Demonstrate cultural sensitivity
- Use appropriate assessment techniques
- Prioritize assessment findings

Documentation Accuracy Evaluation

Your documentation will be assessed for:

- Completeness of information
- Accuracy of findings
- Appropriate use of medical terminology
- Proper formatting and organization
- Timeliness of documentation
- Legal and ethical compliance
- Integration with plan of care

Peer Evaluation of Interview Techniques

Your classmates will evaluate your:

- Communication skills
- Therapeutic relationship building
- Cultural sensitivity
- Active listening abilities
- Appropriate questioning techniques
- Professional boundaries
- Empathy and compassion

Competency Checklist: Complete Head-to-Toe Assessment

Demonstrate competency in:

- Health history collection
- General survey and vital signs
- Head and neck assessment
- Cardiac assessment
- Respiratory assessment
- Abdominal assessment
- Neurological assessment
- Musculoskeletal assessment
- Skin assessment
- Documentation of findings

Moving Forward with Confidence

Health assessment is the foundation of all nursing care. Every intervention you perform, every decision you make, and every outcome you achieve begins with thorough, thoughtful assessment. As you develop these skills, remember that assessment is not just about gathering data—it's about understanding the whole person and building therapeutic relationships that promote healing.

The techniques you've learned in this chapter will serve you throughout your nursing career. Whether you're working in a busy emergency department, a quiet medical unit, or a patient's home, these assessment skills will help you provide safe, effective care. Practice regularly, seek feedback from experienced nurses, and always remember that behind every assessment is a person who needs your expertise, compassion, and care.

In the next chapter, we'll explore how to use your assessment skills to identify and prevent infections—one of the most important aspects of patient safety in healthcare.

Key Takeaways

1. **Assessment is the foundation of all nursing care.** Every intervention, decision, and outcome begins with thorough, systematic assessment.
2. **Cultural competence enhances assessment accuracy.** Understanding patients' cultural backgrounds helps you provide more effective, respectful care.
3. **Therapeutic communication builds trust and gathers better information.** Your communication skills are as important as your technical skills.
4. **Physical assessment techniques require practice and confidence.** Regular practice helps you develop the skills needed for accurate assessment.
5. **Vital signs provide crucial information about patient status.** Understanding normal variations and accurate measurement techniques is essential.

6. **Documentation must be accurate, complete, and timely.**
   Good documentation protects patients, providers, and
   healthcare organizations.
7. **Electronic health records offer advantages but require
   careful use.** Understanding EHR systems helps you provide
   safer, more efficient care.

Chapter 4: Infection Control and Safety

Every healthcare worker carries an invisible responsibility that weighs more than any stethoscope or medication they might hold. With every patient interaction, every procedure performed, and every surface touched, you have the power to either spread infection or stop it in its tracks. This responsibility isn't just about following rules—it's about understanding that you stand between vulnerable patients and potentially life-threatening organisms.

Healthcare-associated infections affect 1 in 31 hospital patients on any given day, resulting in tens of thousands of deaths annually (22). But here's the remarkable part: most of these infections are preventable. The simple act of washing your hands, wearing protective equipment correctly, and following established protocols can literally save lives.

Patient safety extends far beyond infection control. It includes fall prevention, medication safety, patient identification, and creating environments where healing can occur. As a nurse, you'll be the last line of defense against errors, the first to notice potential problems, and the advocate who speaks up when something isn't right.

Infection Prevention Fundamentals

Chain of Infection

Understanding how infections spread is like understanding how a chain works—break any link, and the whole chain falls apart. The chain of infection consists of six essential elements that must all be present for infection to occur (23).

Infectious agent is the microorganism that causes disease. These can be bacteria, viruses, fungi, or parasites. Each type has different characteristics:

- **Bacteria** like Staphylococcus aureus or Escherichia coli can multiply rapidly in the right conditions

- **Viruses** such as influenza or COVID-19 require living cells to reproduce
- **Fungi** including Candida species can cause serious infections in immunocompromised patients
- **Parasites** like malaria or intestinal worms can cause chronic infections

Reservoir is where the microorganism lives and multiplies. Common reservoirs include:

- Human sources (patients, healthcare workers, visitors)
- Environmental sources (water, soil, surfaces)
- Animal sources (pets, wildlife, livestock)
- Inanimate objects (medical equipment, linens, food)

Portal of exit is how the microorganism leaves the reservoir:

- Respiratory tract (coughing, sneezing, talking)
- Gastrointestinal tract (vomiting, diarrhea)
- Genitourinary tract (urination, sexual contact)
- Blood and other body fluids (wounds, injections)
- Skin and mucous membranes (direct contact)

Mode of transmission describes how the microorganism moves from one place to another:

- **Contact transmission** (direct or indirect touch)
- **Droplet transmission** (large particles that travel short distances)
- **Airborne transmission** (small particles that remain suspended in air)
- **Vector transmission** (insects or animals that carry organisms)
- **Vehicle transmission** (contaminated food, water, or objects)

Portal of entry is how the microorganism enters a new host:

- Respiratory tract (inhalation)
- Gastrointestinal tract (ingestion)
- Genitourinary tract (sexual contact, catheterization)

- Blood and other body fluids (injections, transfusions)
- Skin and mucous membranes (breaks in skin barrier)

Susceptible host is a person who lacks resistance to the microorganism. Risk factors include:

- Weakened immune system
- Chronic diseases
- Malnutrition
- Stress
- Age (very young or very old)
- Medications that suppress immunity

Interactive Exercise: Chain of Infection Puzzle Activity

Create a puzzle activity to reinforce understanding of the infection chain:

Materials needed:

- Six puzzle pieces representing each link in the chain
- Various scenario cards describing different infections
- Intervention cards showing how to break each link

Instructions:

1. Assemble the complete chain of infection puzzle
2. Select a scenario card (e.g., "Hospital patient develops pneumonia")
3. Identify all six links in the chain for that scenario
4. Choose intervention cards that could break each link
5. Discuss which interventions are most practical and effective

Example scenario: Healthcare worker develops influenza

- **Infectious agent:** Influenza virus
- **Reservoir:** Infected patient
- **Portal of exit:** Respiratory tract (coughing)
- **Mode of transmission:** Droplet transmission

- **Portal of entry:** Respiratory tract (inhalation)
- **Susceptible host:** Unvaccinated healthcare worker

Possible interventions:

- Antiviral medications (reduce infectious agent)
- Isolation of infected patients (control reservoir)
- Respiratory etiquette (block portal of exit)
- Physical distancing (interrupt transmission)
- Masks and eye protection (protect portal of entry)
- Influenza vaccination (protect susceptible host)

This exercise helps students understand that multiple interventions can be used simultaneously to prevent infection.

Hand Hygiene Excellence

Hand hygiene is the single most important measure to prevent healthcare-associated infections (24). Yet compliance rates among healthcare workers often fall below 50%. Understanding the science behind hand hygiene and developing consistent habits can dramatically improve patient safety.

CDC/WHO guidelines provide evidence-based recommendations for hand hygiene:

- Use alcohol-based hand rub for routine decontamination
- Wash hands with soap and water when visibly soiled
- Perform hand hygiene before and after patient contact
- Use proper technique for both hand washing and hand rub application
- Maintain short, clean fingernails
- Avoid artificial nails and nail polish in clinical areas

Five moments for hand hygiene identify critical times when hand hygiene is essential (25):

1. **Before patient contact** to protect the patient from organisms on your hands

2. **Before aseptic procedures** to prevent organisms from entering sterile sites
3. **After body fluid exposure** to protect yourself from patient organisms
4. **After patient contact** to protect yourself and prevent cross-contamination
5. **After contact with patient surroundings** to prevent contamination from environment

Proper technique demonstration ensures effectiveness:

Alcohol-based hand rub technique:

1. Apply product to palm of one hand
2. Rub hands together, covering all surfaces
3. Rub between fingers and around thumbs
4. Rub fingertips against opposite palms
5. Continue until hands are dry (15-20 seconds)

Handwashing technique:

1. Wet hands with water
2. Apply soap and lather thoroughly
3. Scrub all surfaces for at least 20 seconds
4. Rinse thoroughly with water
5. Dry with disposable towel
6. Use towel to turn off faucet

Practical Exercise: Glow-in-the-Dark Hand Hygiene Evaluation

Use fluorescent lotion and ultraviolet light to demonstrate hand hygiene effectiveness:

Setup:

- Apply fluorescent lotion to represent "germs" on hands
- Attempt hand hygiene using usual technique
- Use UV light to reveal missed areas
- Repeat with improved technique until all "germs" are removed

Common missed areas:

- Thumbs and thumb webs
- Fingertips and under nails
- Backs of hands
- Wrists
- Between fingers

Learning outcomes:

- Visual demonstration of hand hygiene effectiveness
- Identification of commonly missed areas
- Motivation to improve technique
- Understanding of proper timing

Assessment Tool: Hand Hygiene Compliance Checklist

Use this checklist to evaluate hand hygiene practices:

Timing (Did the person perform hand hygiene?):

- Before patient contact
- Before aseptic procedures
- After body fluid exposure
- After patient contact
- After contact with patient surroundings

Technique (Was proper technique used?):

- Appropriate product selected
- Adequate amount of product used
- All hand surfaces covered
- Proper duration maintained
- Hands completely dry before patient contact

Compliance score: (Number of appropriate actions / Total opportunities) × 100

Regular monitoring and feedback help improve compliance rates and patient safety.

Standard Precautions

Standard precautions are the foundation of infection control in healthcare. They're called "standard" because they should be used with every patient, every time, regardless of diagnosis or suspected infection status.

When to implement: Standard precautions apply to all patient care activities involving:

- Blood and all body fluids (except sweat)
- Secretions and excretions
- Non-intact skin
- Mucous membranes

Components of standard precautions include:

- Hand hygiene before and after patient contact
- Personal protective equipment when indicated
- Safe injection practices
- Respiratory hygiene and cough etiquette
- Safe handling of contaminated equipment
- Environmental cleaning and disinfection

Body substance isolation means treating all body fluids as potentially infectious. This approach protects both patients and healthcare workers from known and unknown infections.

Case Study: Emergency Department Triage Decisions

Sarah, an emergency department nurse, faces multiple infection control challenges during a busy shift. Her decisions demonstrate how standard precautions protect everyone in the healthcare environment.

Patient 1: A 45-year-old construction worker arrives with a laceration on his forearm from a rusty nail. The wound is bleeding actively, and his clothes are dirty from the construction site.

Sarah's response:

- Applies standard precautions immediately
- Dons gloves before examining the wound
- Uses eye protection due to risk of splashing
- Covers the wound with sterile dressing
- Ensures tetanus vaccination is current
- Disposes of contaminated materials properly

Patient 2: A 25-year-old woman presents with fever, cough, and difficulty breathing. She mentions that several coworkers have been ill recently.

Sarah's response:

- Immediately places surgical mask on patient
- Moves patient to negative pressure room
- Dons N95 respirator for close contact
- Implements droplet precautions in addition to standard precautions
- Notifies physician about possible respiratory infection
- Ensures all staff use appropriate PPE

Patient 3: An elderly man arrives by ambulance, confused and incontinent. His family reports he's been having diarrhea for several days.

Sarah's response:

- Uses standard precautions for all contact
- Dons gloves and gown due to contamination risk
- Considers contact precautions pending diagnosis
- Collects stool specimen for testing
- Ensures proper cleaning of contaminated areas
- Educates family about hand hygiene

Patient 4: A healthcare worker from another hospital seeks treatment for a needlestick injury that occurred 30 minutes ago.

Sarah's response:

- Provides immediate wound care using standard precautions
- Initiates exposure protocol
- Arranges for baseline testing of both source patient and exposed worker
- Coordinates with employee health for follow-up
- Documents incident thoroughly
- Provides counseling and support

These scenarios demonstrate how standard precautions provide a consistent approach to infection control while allowing for additional precautions when needed.

Transmission-Based Precautions

When standard precautions aren't sufficient to prevent transmission, additional precautions are necessary. These transmission-based precautions are designed for patients with known or suspected infections that spread through specific routes.

Contact Precautions

Contact precautions prevent transmission of infections that spread through direct or indirect contact with patients or their environment. These precautions are used for organisms that can survive on surfaces and be transmitted through touch.

Indications and requirements for contact precautions include:

- Multidrug-resistant organisms (MRSA, VRE, CRE)
- Clostridioides difficile infections
- Norovirus and other viral gastroenteritis
- Scabies and other skin infections
- Wound infections with drainage

Proper gowning and gloving follows specific steps:

1. Perform hand hygiene
2. Put on gown, ensuring full coverage
3. Put on gloves, covering gown cuffs
4. Enter patient room
5. Provide patient care
6. Remove PPE in proper sequence
7. Perform hand hygiene

Environmental considerations include:

- Dedicate patient care equipment when possible
- Clean and disinfect shared equipment between patients
- Limit patient movement outside the room
- Ensure adequate cleaning and disinfection of patient room
- Consider cohorting patients with same infection

Skill Station: Donning and Doffing PPE Sequence

Practice the correct sequence for putting on and removing PPE:

Donning sequence:

1. **Hand hygiene** - Clean hands thoroughly
2. **Gown** - Put on gown, tie at neck and waist
3. **Mask or respirator** - Secure over nose and mouth
4. **Eye protection** - Put on goggles or face shield
5. **Gloves** - Put on gloves, extend over gown cuffs

Doffing sequence:

1. **Gloves** - Remove carefully, don't touch outer surface
2. **Gown** - Remove by pulling away from body
3. **Hand hygiene** - Clean hands immediately
4. **Eye protection** - Remove by lifting headband
5. **Mask or respirator** - Remove by lifting bottom ties first
6. **Hand hygiene** - Final hand cleaning

Common mistakes to avoid:

- Touching contaminated surfaces during removal
- Incorrect sequence of removal
- Inadequate hand hygiene
- Reusing disposable equipment
- Touching face or hair during procedure

Droplet and Airborne Precautions

Droplet and airborne precautions protect against infections transmitted through respiratory particles. Understanding the difference between these transmission modes is crucial for selecting appropriate precautions.

Droplet precautions are used for organisms spread through large respiratory particles that don't remain suspended in air:

- Influenza
- Pertussis (whooping cough)
- Streptococcal pharyngitis
- Pneumonic plague
- Rubella

Airborne precautions are used for organisms spread through small particles that remain suspended in air:

- Tuberculosis
- Measles
- Varicella (chickenpox)
- Disseminated herpes zoster
- SARS and other emerging respiratory pathogens

Disease-specific requirements vary based on transmission mode:

- **Droplet:** Surgical mask, private room preferred
- **Airborne:** N95 respirator, negative pressure room required

N95 respirator fit testing ensures proper protection:

- Annual fit testing required
- Qualitative or quantitative testing methods
- Multiple sizes and models available
- Proper seal check before each use
- Medical clearance required

Negative pressure rooms create airflow that prevents contaminated air from escaping:

- Air changes per hour: minimum 6 for existing facilities, 12 for new construction
- Air exhausted directly outside or through HEPA filtration
- Door must remain closed
- Pressure monitoring required

Simulation: Managing Tuberculosis Patient Admission

Practice managing a high-risk airborne infection:

Scenario: A 35-year-old man presents to the emergency department with a 3-week history of cough, fever, night sweats, and weight loss. He recently immigrated from a country with high tuberculosis prevalence.

Immediate actions:

1. Place surgical mask on patient immediately
2. Move patient to negative pressure room
3. Notify physician and infection control
4. Don N95 respirator for close contact
5. Limit number of staff entering room
6. Ensure all visitors wear appropriate PPE

Ongoing management:

- Collect sputum specimens for testing
- Initiate contact investigation
- Ensure proper isolation until diagnosis confirmed
- Provide patient education about isolation

- Monitor for treatment compliance
- Coordinate with public health authorities

Key learning points:

- Recognition of high-risk symptoms
- Importance of immediate isolation
- Proper PPE selection and use
- Multidisciplinary coordination
- Public health implications

Isolation Protocols

Isolation can be psychologically challenging for patients and families. Understanding the emotional impact and providing appropriate support is essential for comprehensive care.

Patient education and support helps patients understand and cope with isolation:

- Explain the reason for isolation in simple terms
- Provide written information about precautions
- Discuss expected duration of isolation
- Address concerns and answer questions
- Involve family in education when appropriate

Visitor management balances infection control with psychosocial needs:

- Limit number of visitors when possible
- Provide instruction on PPE use
- Ensure visitors understand precautions
- Consider alternatives like video calling
- Support visitor emotional needs

Psychological effects of isolation can include:

- Anxiety and depression
- Feelings of abandonment

- Anger and frustration
- Social isolation
- Reduced sense of control

Case Study: Pediatric Patient in Isolation - Family Support Strategies

Five-year-old Emma is admitted with respiratory syncytial virus (RSV) and requires droplet precautions. Her parents are anxious about the isolation requirements and worry about Emma's emotional well-being.

Challenges identified:

- Emma is frightened by masked healthcare workers
- Parents feel helpless and confused about precautions
- Emma's siblings cannot visit due to infection risk
- Family cultural practices emphasize community support
- Emma's normal routines are disrupted

Nursing interventions:

1. **Education and communication:**
   - Explain isolation in age-appropriate terms
   - Use pictures and simple language
   - Demonstrate proper hand hygiene
   - Provide written materials in family's language
2. **Emotional support:**
   - Spend extra time with Emma during procedures
   - Encourage parents to stay with Emma
   - Facilitate video calls with siblings
   - Provide age-appropriate activities and toys
3. **Cultural considerations:**
   - Understand family's cultural beliefs about illness
   - Adapt isolation procedures when possible
   - Respect religious or cultural practices
   - Involve cultural liaisons if available
4. **Family involvement:**
   - Teach parents proper PPE use

      o Encourage parents to participate in care
      o Provide emotional support for parents
      o Connect family with social services if needed

5. **Continuity of care:**
   - Assign consistent nursing staff when possible
   - Maintain familiar routines
   - Coordinate with child life specialists
   - Plan for smooth transition to home care

Outcomes:

- Emma's anxiety decreases with consistent caregivers
- Parents feel more confident about managing isolation
- Family maintains connections through technology
- Emma's recovery proceeds without complications
- Family expresses satisfaction with care received

This case illustrates how thoughtful nursing care can minimize the negative effects of isolation while maintaining safety.

Patient Safety Essentials

Patient Identification

Patient identification errors can lead to serious harm, including wrong-site surgery, medication errors, and inappropriate treatments. Reliable identification systems are essential for patient safety.

Two-identifier requirement is the standard for patient identification:

- Patient's name
- Date of birth
- Medical record number
- Assigned identification number

Never use:

- Room number

- Bed number
- Diagnosis
- Age alone

Barcode scanning systems provide additional safety:

- Scan patient wristband before procedures
- Verify match with medication or treatment
- Alert system for mismatches
- Backup procedures when system fails

Wrong patient errors prevention strategies include:

- Always ask patient to state name and date of birth
- Check identification band before every interaction
- Verify identification with family when appropriate
- Use two identifiers consistently
- Address patients by name during care

Practical Exercise: Patient Identification Scenarios

Practice proper identification in various situations:

Scenario 1: Emergency department

- Unconscious patient arrives by ambulance
- No identification available
- Multiple patients with similar names
- Family members present

Scenario 2: Pediatric unit

- Young child unable to state name
- Parent not present
- Multiple children in same room
- Identification band removed by child

Scenario 3: Surgical suite

- Patient sedated for procedure
- Multiple procedures scheduled
- Similar patient names
- Time pressure to begin surgery

Scenario 4: Home health

- Patient with dementia
- Multiple medications to administer
- Family caregiver present
- No hospital identification band

Each scenario requires adaptation of identification procedures while maintaining safety standards.

Fall Prevention

Falls are among the most common adverse events in healthcare settings. Understanding risk factors and implementing prevention strategies can significantly reduce fall-related injuries.

Fall risk assessment tools help identify high-risk patients:

- **Morse Fall Scale** assesses history of falls, secondary diagnosis, ambulatory aid, IV/heparin lock, gait, and mental status
- **STRATIFY** evaluates recent falls, agitation, visual impairment, toileting urgency, and transfer/mobility issues
- **Hendrich II Fall Risk Model** includes confusion, depression, altered elimination, dizziness, male gender, antiepileptics, and benzodiazepines

Environmental modifications reduce fall risk:

- Keep bed in lowest position
- Ensure adequate lighting
- Remove clutter from walkways
- Use non-slip footwear
- Install grab bars in bathrooms

- Keep call bell within reach

Patient and family education promotes safety awareness:

- Explain fall risk factors
- Demonstrate safe transfer techniques
- Encourage asking for help
- Discuss medication effects
- Review home safety measures

Progressive Skill: Develop Individualized Fall Prevention Plans

Create comprehensive fall prevention plans for different patient populations:

Plan 1: Older adult with multiple medications

- Review medication effects on balance
- Implement gradual position changes
- Ensure adequate lighting
- Provide assistive devices
- Schedule regular toileting

Plan 2: Post-operative patient

- Assess effects of anesthesia
- Monitor for orthostatic changes
- Provide pain management
- Ensure proper ambulation assistance
- Educate about activity restrictions

Plan 3: Patient with neurological condition

- Assess cognitive function
- Modify environment for safety
- Provide constant observation if needed
- Use bed alarms appropriately
- Coordinate with rehabilitation team

Plan 4: Pediatric patient

- Age-appropriate safety measures
- Parent/caregiver education
- Secure medical equipment
- Provide appropriate supervision
- Use safety devices as needed

Each plan should be individualized based on specific risk factors and patient needs.

Safe Patient Handling

Manual patient handling is a leading cause of injury among healthcare workers. Understanding body mechanics and using assistive devices protects both patients and caregivers.

Body mechanics principles reduce injury risk:

- Keep back straight and neutral
- Bend knees, not back
- Keep load close to body
- Avoid twisting motions
- Use leg muscles for lifting
- Get help for heavy loads

Assistive devices and equipment improve safety:

- Mechanical lifts for dependent patients
- Transfer boards for lateral transfers
- Gait belts for ambulation assistance
- Slide sheets for repositioning
- Standing aids for partial weight-bearing

Transfer techniques vary based on patient condition:

- **Bed to chair:** Assess patient's ability to assist
- **Chair to bed:** Use proper body mechanics
- **Lateral transfer:** Use appropriate equipment

- **Shower transfer:** Ensure adequate assistance

Hands-on Practice: Patient Transfer Laboratory

Practice safe transfer techniques in controlled environment:

Station 1: Bed to wheelchair transfer

- Assess patient's ability to assist
- Position wheelchair appropriately
- Use gait belt for safety
- Provide clear instructions
- Maintain stability throughout transfer

Station 2: Lateral transfer using slide board

- Position equipment correctly
- Ensure adequate staffing
- Use smooth, coordinated movements
- Maintain patient dignity
- Monitor for adverse reactions

Station 3: Mechanical lift operation

- Inspect equipment before use
- Position sling correctly
- Follow manufacturer's instructions
- Ensure patient comfort
- Maintain safety throughout procedure

Station 4: Ambulation assistance

- Assess patient's stability
- Use appropriate assistive devices
- Provide physical support as needed
- Monitor for fatigue or dizziness
- Ensure safe return to bed or chair

Regular practice helps develop competence and confidence in safe patient handling.

Medication Safety

Rights of Medication Administration

Medication errors are among the most common types of errors in healthcare. Understanding and consistently applying the rights of medication administration helps prevent these potentially serious errors.

Traditional 5 rights:

1. **Right patient** - Verify identity using two identifiers
2. **Right medication** - Compare with physician order
3. **Right dose** - Calculate and verify amount
4. **Right route** - Confirm method of administration
5. **Right time** - Administer at prescribed intervals

Additional rights enhance safety: 6. **Right documentation** - Record administration accurately 7. **Right to refuse** - Respect patient's autonomy 8. **Right assessment** - Evaluate patient condition 9. **Right education** - Teach patient about medication 10. **Right evaluation** - Monitor for therapeutic effect

Activity: Medication Error Case Analysis

Review real medication error cases to understand contributing factors:

Case 1: Dosage error

- Patient received 10 units of insulin instead of 1 unit
- Contributing factors: Illegible handwriting, no verification
- Prevention strategies: Electronic prescribing, double-check system
- Lessons learned: Importance of clear communication

Case 2: Wrong patient error

- Patient received medication intended for roommate
- Contributing factors: Inadequate identification, similar names
- Prevention strategies: Two-identifier verification, barcode scanning
- Lessons learned: Never assume patient identity

Case 3: Route error

- IV medication given orally
- Contributing factors: Look-alike packaging, inadequate labeling
- Prevention strategies: Clear labeling, separate storage
- Lessons learned: Importance of reading labels carefully

Case 4: Time error

- Medication given 12 hours early
- Contributing factors: Confusion about schedule, poor communication
- Prevention strategies: Clear scheduling, medication reconciliation
- Lessons learned: Importance of systematic approach

Each case analysis should include:

- Description of the error
- Contributing factors
- Potential consequences
- Prevention strategies
- Lessons learned

High-Alert Medications

High-alert medications have increased risk of causing significant harm when used in error. These medications require special safety measures and heightened awareness.

ISMP high-alert drug list includes medications such as:

- Insulin and oral hypoglycemics
- Anticoagulants (warfarin, heparin)
- Opioid analgesics
- Chemotherapy agents
- Neuromuscular blocking agents
- Concentrated electrolytes

Double-check procedures provide additional verification:

- Two nurses independently verify calculations
- Check original order against prepared medication
- Confirm patient identity and appropriateness
- Document both nurses' verification
- Use standardized protocols

Look-alike/sound-alike drugs require special attention:

- Separate storage when possible
- Use tall man lettering (e.g., DOPamine vs. DOBUTamine)
- Implement confirmation procedures
- Educate staff about similar medications
- Use technology alerts when available

Simulation: Insulin Administration Safety

Practice safe insulin administration in realistic scenarios:

Scenario setup:

- Patient with diabetes requiring insulin
- Multiple insulin types available
- Sliding scale orders
- Blood glucose monitoring required
- Potential for calculation errors

Safety measures practiced:

- Verify patient identity using two identifiers
- Check blood glucose before administration
- Calculate dose using sliding scale
- Have second nurse verify calculation
- Use insulin syringe appropriate for concentration
- Administer at correct time and route
- Document administration accurately
- Monitor patient for hypoglycemia

Learning objectives:

- Understand insulin types and actions
- Practice safe calculation methods
- Recognize signs of hypoglycemia
- Implement double-check procedures
- Use technology safely

Debriefing points:

- Discuss near-misses or errors
- Review prevention strategies
- Identify system improvements
- Reinforce importance of vigilance
- Plan for continuous improvement

Chapter 4 Skills Assessment

Your competency in infection control and safety can be evaluated through multiple comprehensive methods:

Infection Control OSCE Stations

You'll demonstrate competency in:

- Hand hygiene technique and timing
- Proper PPE donning and doffing
- Standard precautions implementation
- Transmission-based precautions

- Environmental cleaning procedures
- Waste disposal protocols

PPE Competency Demonstration

Your skills will be assessed for:

- Correct sequence of PPE application
- Proper fit and coverage
- Safe removal techniques
- Appropriate disposal methods
- Hand hygiene compliance
- Adaptation to different scenarios

Safety Audit of Simulated Patient Room

You'll evaluate a patient room for:

- Fall risk hazards
- Infection control compliance
- Equipment safety
- Environmental cleanliness
- Patient identification systems
- Emergency equipment accessibility

Critical Thinking: Outbreak Management Scenario

You'll analyze a simulated outbreak situation:

- Identify potential sources and modes of transmission
- Recommend appropriate isolation precautions
- Develop staff education plans
- Coordinate with infection control team
- Implement prevention strategies
- Monitor effectiveness of interventions

Building a Culture of Safety

Infection control and patient safety aren't just individual responsibilities—they're organizational commitments that require everyone's participation. As you develop your skills, remember that every action you take can either contribute to safety or create risk. The habits you develop now will serve you throughout your career and protect the patients who trust you with their care.

Safety culture thrives when healthcare workers feel empowered to speak up about concerns, report errors without fear of punishment, and continuously look for ways to improve. As a new nurse, you bring fresh eyes and perspectives that can help identify problems and solutions that others might miss.

In the next chapter, we'll explore medication administration—one of the most important and potentially dangerous aspects of nursing practice. The safety principles you've learned here will provide the foundation for safe medication practices throughout your career.

Key Takeaways

1. **Infection control is everyone's responsibility.** Understanding the chain of infection and how to break it protects patients, healthcare workers, and visitors.
2. **Hand hygiene is the most important infection control measure.** Proper technique and timing can prevent most healthcare-associated infections.
3. **Standard precautions apply to all patients.** Treat all body fluids as potentially infectious and use appropriate protective measures.
4. **Transmission-based precautions require additional safety measures.** Understanding different transmission modes helps you select appropriate precautions.
5. **Patient identification prevents serious errors.** Always use two identifiers and verify patient identity before every intervention.
6. **Fall prevention requires comprehensive assessment and intervention.** Individual risk factors guide personalized prevention plans.

7. **Medication safety depends on systematic approaches.** The rights of medication administration provide a framework for safe practice.
8. **High-alert medications require special precautions.** Double-check procedures and heightened awareness prevent serious errors.

Chapter 5: Medication Administration

In your hands rests a small white tablet that weighs less than a gram. To anyone else, it might look insignificant—just another pill among thousands dispensed daily in healthcare facilities worldwide. But you know better. You understand that this seemingly simple medication represents the culmination of years of research, careful prescribing, and now, your skilled administration. You know that giving this medication correctly could ease someone's pain, slow the progression of disease, or even save a life. You also know that a single error could cause harm.

Medication administration is one of the most complex and high-stakes responsibilities in nursing. Every year, nurses safely administer billions of doses of medications, but the potential for error always exists. According to the Institute of Medicine, medication errors harm at least 1.5 million people annually in the United States alone (26). Yet most of these errors are preventable through systematic approaches, careful attention to detail, and thorough understanding of pharmacological principles.

As a nurse, you'll be the final checkpoint between a medication order and a patient. Physicians prescribe medications, pharmacists dispense them, but you're the one who puts them directly into patients' bodies. This responsibility requires not just technical skill, but also clinical judgment, critical thinking, and the confidence to speak up when something doesn't seem right.

Pharmacology Foundations

Drug Classifications

Understanding how medications work and how they're organized helps you anticipate effects, recognize adverse reactions, and provide better patient care. Medications are classified in several ways, but the most useful classification for nurses is by therapeutic effect—what the medication does for the patient.

Cardiovascular medications affect heart function and blood circulation:

- **Antihypertensives** lower blood pressure through various mechanisms
- **Antiarrhythmics** regulate heart rhythm
- **Anticoagulants** prevent blood clot formation
- **Diuretics** increase urine production and reduce fluid volume

Respiratory medications affect breathing and lung function:

- **Bronchodilators** open airways in conditions like asthma
- **Mucolytics** thin respiratory secretions
- **Antitussives** suppress coughing
- **Expectorants** help clear mucus from airways

Gastrointestinal medications affect digestion and elimination:

- **Antacids** neutralize stomach acid
- **Proton pump inhibitors** reduce acid production
- **Antiemetics** prevent nausea and vomiting
- **Laxatives** promote bowel movements

Nervous system medications affect brain and nerve function:

- **Analgesics** relieve pain
- **Sedatives** promote relaxation and sleep
- **Anticonvulsants** prevent seizures
- **Antidepressants** treat mood disorders

Endocrine medications affect hormone balance:

- **Insulin** regulates blood sugar
- **Thyroid hormones** regulate metabolism
- **Corticosteroids** reduce inflammation
- **Oral contraceptives** prevent pregnancy

Anti-infective medications fight infections:

- **Antibiotics** kill or inhibit bacteria
- **Antivirals** treat viral infections
- **Antifungals** treat fungal infections
- **Antiparasitics** treat parasitic infections

Study Tool: Drug Classification Flashcards

Create flashcards to learn drug classifications:

Front of card: Medication name (generic and brand) **Back of card:**

- Classification
- Primary indication
- Common side effects
- Nursing considerations
- Patient teaching points

Example card: Front: Metformin (Glucophage) **Back:**

- **Classification:** Antidiabetic (biguanide)
- **Primary indication:** Type 2 diabetes
- **Common side effects:** Gastrointestinal upset, lactic acidosis (rare)
- **Nursing considerations:** Monitor blood glucose, assess kidney function
- **Patient teaching:** Take with food, recognize hypoglycemia signs

Start with 20-30 common medications and gradually expand your collection. Review cards regularly to reinforce learning.

Pharmacokinetics and Pharmacodynamics

Understanding what happens to medications in the body helps you predict effects, timing, and potential problems. Pharmacokinetics describes what the body does to the drug, while pharmacodynamics describes what the drug does to the body.

Absorption is how medications enter the bloodstream:

- **Oral medications** must dissolve and be absorbed through the gastrointestinal tract
- **Intravenous medications** go directly into circulation
- **Topical medications** are absorbed through the skin
- **Inhaled medications** are absorbed through the lungs

Factors affecting absorption include:

- Route of administration
- Blood flow to absorption site
- Presence of food in stomach
- pH of absorption site
- Patient's health status

Distribution is how medications spread throughout the body:

- Medications travel through bloodstream to target tissues
- Protein binding affects availability of active drug
- Blood-brain barrier limits access to brain tissue
- Placental barrier affects fetal exposure

Metabolism is how the body breaks down medications:

- Most metabolism occurs in the liver
- Some medications are metabolized to active compounds
- Genetic variations affect metabolism rates
- Disease states can alter metabolism

Excretion is how medications leave the body:

- Kidneys eliminate most medications
- Lungs eliminate some volatile compounds
- Liver eliminates some medications through bile
- Skin eliminates small amounts through sweat

Drug interactions occur when medications affect each other:

- **Synergistic effects** occur when combined effects are greater than individual effects

98

•

Synergistic effects occur when combined effects are greater than individual effects

- **Antagonistic effects** occur when medications oppose each other
- **Additive effects** occur when medications have similar actions
- **Altered absorption** can occur when medications bind to each other
- **Altered metabolism** can occur when one medication affects another's breakdown

Case Study: Polypharmacy in Elderly Patient

Meet Mrs. Thompson, an 82-year-old woman who takes multiple medications for various chronic conditions. Her case illustrates the complexity of pharmacokinetics and pharmacodynamics in real-world practice.

Mrs. Thompson's medications:

- Warfarin (Coumadin) for atrial fibrillation
- Metformin (Glucophage) for diabetes
- Lisinopril (Prinivil) for hypertension
- Furosemide (Lasix) for heart failure
- Omeprazole (Prilosec) for acid reflux
- Calcium carbonate (Tums) for bone health

Pharmacokinetic considerations:

- **Absorption:** Omeprazole may affect absorption of other medications by changing stomach pH

- **Distribution:** Warfarin is highly protein-bound, so changes in protein levels affect drug activity
- **Metabolism:** Age-related liver changes may slow metabolism of warfarin and other drugs
- **Excretion:** Kidney function decline affects elimination of metformin and furosemide

Potential drug interactions:

- Calcium may bind to other medications, reducing their absorption
- Furosemide may increase warfarin effects by displacing it from protein binding sites
- Omeprazole may affect warfarin metabolism, requiring dose adjustments

Nursing implications:

- Monitor for signs of bleeding due to warfarin interactions
- Check kidney function before giving metformin
- Separate calcium administration from other medications
- Monitor blood pressure and electrolytes with furosemide
- Assess for signs of hypoglycemia with metformin

Patient education priorities:

- Importance of taking medications as prescribed
- Recognition of bleeding signs with warfarin
- Proper timing of medication administration
- When to contact healthcare provider
- Importance of regular monitoring

This case demonstrates how understanding pharmacokinetics and pharmacodynamics helps nurses provide safer, more effective medication administration.

Dosage Calculations

Basic Math Review

Accurate dosage calculations are essential for patient safety. Most medication errors involve dosage calculation mistakes, making mathematical competence a critical nursing skill.

Fractions represent parts of a whole:

- **Proper fractions:** Numerator is smaller than denominator (3/4)
- **Improper fractions:** Numerator is larger than denominator (5/3)
- **Mixed numbers:** Whole number plus fraction (2 1/2)

Decimals are another way to express parts of a whole:

- **Place values:** Tenths (0.1), hundredths (0.01), thousandths (0.001)
- **Converting fractions to decimals:** Divide numerator by denominator
- **Rounding:** Round to appropriate decimal places for accuracy

Percentages express parts of 100:

- **Converting percentages to decimals:** Move decimal point two places left
- **Converting decimals to percentages:** Move decimal point two places right
- **Common medical percentages:** 0.9% normal saline, 5% dextrose

Metric system conversions are essential for medication calculations:

- **Length:** Meter (m), centimeter (cm), millimeter (mm)
- **Weight:** Kilogram (kg), gram (g), milligram (mg), microgram (mcg)
- **Volume:** Liter (L), milliliter (mL), cubic centimeter (cc)

Practice Problems: Progressive Difficulty Calculations

Level 1: Basic conversions

1. Convert 2.5 g to mg
2. Convert 500 mL to L
3. Convert 0.25 mg to mcg
4. Convert 1500 mL to L

Level 2: Simple dosage calculations

1. Order: 250 mg. Available: 500 mg tablets. How many tablets?
2. Order: 0.5 g. Available: 250 mg capsules. How many capsules?
3. Order: 15 mL. Available: 5 mL/dose. How many doses?

Level 3: Complex calculations

1. Order: 10 mg/kg. Patient weighs 70 kg. Total dose?
2. Order: 500 mg in 100 mL over 30 minutes. What is the flow rate?
3. Order: 2 units/kg/hr. Patient weighs 80 kg. Units per hour?

Level 4: Critical care calculations

1. Dopamine 400 mg in 250 mL at 10 mcg/kg/min for 70 kg patient
2. Insulin drip: 100 units in 100 mL, start at 2 units/hr
3. Heparin protocol: 80 units/kg bolus, then 18 units/kg/hr

Dosage Calculation Methods

Different calculation methods work better for different people and situations. Learning multiple methods provides flexibility and helps verify answers.

Dimensional analysis uses conversion factors to solve problems:

- Set up equation with desired units
- Use conversion factors to cancel unwanted units

- Multiply across numerators and denominators
- Solve for final answer

Example: Order: 0.5 g. Available: 250 mg tablets. How many tablets?

0.5 g × (1000 mg/1 g) × (1 tablet/250 mg) = 2 tablets

Ratio and proportion sets up equivalent relationships:

- Known ratio : Unknown ratio
- Cross multiply to solve
- Check answer for reasonableness

Example: Order: 250 mg. Available: 500 mg in 2 tablets. How many tablets?

500 mg : 2 tablets = 250 mg : x tablets 500x = 500 x = 1 tablet

Formula method uses a standard equation:

- Desired dose/Available dose × Quantity = Amount to give
- Simple and straightforward for basic calculations
- May need modification for complex problems

Example: Order: 0.25 mg. Available: 0.5 mg/tablet. How many tablets?

0.25 mg/0.5 mg × 1 tablet = 0.5 tablet

Interactive Game: Dosage Calculation Competition

Create a game-based learning environment to practice calculations:

Setup:

- Divide class into teams
- Prepare calculation problems of varying difficulty

- Use buzzers or raise hands for answers
- Award points for correct answers
- Include bonus rounds for complex problems

Game categories:

- Basic conversions (1 point each)
- Simple dosage calculations (2 points each)
- IV flow rate calculations (3 points each)
- Critical care calculations (5 points each)
- Pediatric calculations (5 points each)

Sample problems:

- **Basic:** Convert 2.5 L to mL
- **Simple:** Order 500 mg, available 250 mg tablets
- **IV calculation:** 1000 mL over 8 hours, drop factor 15
- **Critical care:** Dopamine 5 mcg/kg/min for 80 kg patient
- **Pediatric:** Acetaminophen 15 mg/kg for 25 kg child

Benefits of game format:

- Increases engagement and motivation
- Provides immediate feedback
- Encourages teamwork and discussion
- Reduces anxiety about calculations
- Makes learning enjoyable

Pediatric and Weight-Based Dosing

Pediatric medication administration requires special considerations because children aren't just small adults. Their physiology, metabolism, and responses to medications differ significantly from adults.

Body Surface Area (BSA) calculations provide more accurate dosing for children:

- BSA accounts for height and weight

- More accurate than weight alone for many medications
- Calculated using nomograms or formulas
- Expressed in square meters (m²)

Mosteller formula: BSA = √(height in cm × weight in kg)/3600

Safe dose ranges help verify appropriate pediatric doses:

- Always check recommended pediatric dose range
- Calculate dose based on child's weight or BSA
- Compare calculated dose to safe range
- Question orders outside safe parameters

Case Scenarios: Pediatric Medication Calculations

Scenario 1: Acetaminophen for fever

- Patient: 3-year-old, 15 kg
- Order: Acetaminophen 15 mg/kg PO q6h PRN fever
- Available: 160 mg/5 mL suspension
- Calculate: 15 mg/kg × 15 kg = 225 mg per dose
- Volume: 225 mg × (5 mL/160 mg) = 7.03 mL per dose

Scenario 2: Antibiotic for infection

- Patient: 8-year-old, 25 kg
- Order: Amoxicillin 20 mg/kg PO q8h
- Available: 250 mg/5 mL suspension
- Calculate: 20 mg/kg × 25 kg = 500 mg per dose
- Volume: 500 mg × (5 mL/250 mg) = 10 mL per dose

Scenario 3: IV medication for seizure

- Patient: 6-month-old, 8 kg
- Order: Phenobarbital 20 mg/kg IV loading dose
- Available: 65 mg/mL injection
- Calculate: 20 mg/kg × 8 kg = 160 mg total dose
- Volume: 160 mg × (1 mL/65 mg) = 2.46 mL

Safety considerations:

- Double-check all pediatric calculations
- Verify dose against reference ranges
- Consider developmental factors
- Use appropriate measuring devices
- Monitor for side effects carefully

Medication Administration Routes

Oral Medications

Oral administration is the most common and convenient route for medications. However, it requires understanding of absorption factors and proper techniques to ensure safety and effectiveness.

Tablet administration considerations:

- Check for scored tablets before crushing
- Some tablets have enteric coatings that shouldn't be broken
- Extended-release formulations must remain intact
- Use pill crusher only when appropriate

Liquid administration requires accuracy:

- Use calibrated measuring devices
- Shake suspensions before measuring
- Check expiration dates of opened liquids
- Store according to manufacturer instructions

Sublingual medications dissolve under the tongue:

- Don't give with water
- Patient shouldn't eat or drink until dissolved
- Common example: nitroglycerin for chest pain
- Rapid absorption and onset of action

Crushing medications safely when necessary:

- Check references for crush-safe medications
- Use appropriate crushing devices
- Mix with small amount of soft food if needed
- Give immediately after crushing
- Clean equipment between patients

Enteral tube medications require special considerations:

- Use liquid formulations when possible
- Crush only crush-safe tablets
- Dissolve in appropriate amount of water
- Flush tube before and after medication
- Check for drug-nutrient interactions

Skill Practice: Medication Preparation and Administration

Practice oral medication administration with various scenarios:

Station 1: Tablet preparation

- Practice identifying crushable vs. non-crushable tablets
- Use pill splitter for scored tablets
- Demonstrate proper crushing technique
- Show correct disposal of unused portions

Station 2: Liquid measurement

- Use various measuring devices (syringes, cups, spoons)
- Practice accurate measurement techniques
- Demonstrate proper pouring at eye level
- Show correct technique for viscous liquids

Station 3: Sublingual administration

- Practice patient education about sublingual route
- Demonstrate proper placement technique
- Explain importance of not swallowing
- Show correct storage of sublingual medications

Station 4: Enteral tube administration

- Practice liquid preparation for tube administration
- Demonstrate proper tube flushing technique
- Show correct medication mixing procedures
- Practice checking tube placement

Injectable Medications

Injectable medications bypass the gastrointestinal tract and often have rapid onset of action. Understanding different injection routes and proper techniques is essential for safe administration.

Intradermal injections are given into the dermis:

- Common uses: allergy testing, tuberculin skin test
- Injection sites: inner forearm, upper back
- Needle: 25-27 gauge, 1/4 to 1/2 inch
- Angle: 10-15 degrees
- Volume: 0.1 mL or less

Subcutaneous injections are given into subcutaneous tissue:

- Common uses: insulin, heparin, vaccines
- Injection sites: abdomen, thigh, upper arm
- Needle: 25-27 gauge, 3/8 to 5/8 inch
- Angle: 45-90 degrees depending on patient size
- Volume: 0.5-1 mL maximum

Intramuscular injections are given into muscle tissue:

- Common uses: vaccines, antibiotics, pain medications
- Injection sites: deltoid, vastus lateralis, ventrogluteal
- Needle: 20-25 gauge, 1 to 1.5 inches
- Angle: 90 degrees
- Volume: up to 3 mL in large muscles

Z-track technique prevents medication leakage:

- Used for medications that can stain tissue
- Pull skin to one side before insertion
- Inject medication slowly
- Wait 10 seconds before withdrawing
- Release skin after needle removal

Needle safety and disposal prevents needlestick injuries:

- Use safety needles when available
- Never recap needles
- Dispose immediately in sharps container
- Don't overfill sharps containers
- Report needlestick injuries immediately

Simulation Lab: Injection Practice on Mannequins

Practice injection techniques in safe environment:

Station 1: Intradermal injection

- Practice proper needle insertion angle
- Observe wheal formation
- Demonstrate proper documentation
- Show correct reading of skin tests

Station 2: Subcutaneous injection

- Practice site selection and rotation
- Demonstrate proper needle insertion
- Show correct technique for insulin administration
- Practice disposal procedures

Station 3: Intramuscular injection

- Practice landmark identification
- Demonstrate proper needle length selection
- Show Z-track technique
- Practice aspiration technique (when indicated)

Station 4: Needle safety

- Practice using safety needles
- Demonstrate proper disposal technique
- Show correct handling of sharps containers
- Practice needlestick injury response

Assessment Tool: Injection Technique Checklist

Evaluate injection competency using standardized criteria:

Preparation:

- Verifies medication order
- Checks patient identity
- Gathers appropriate supplies
- Performs hand hygiene
- Prepares medication correctly

Administration:

- Selects appropriate site
- Uses proper body mechanics
- Inserts needle at correct angle
- Injects medication at appropriate rate
- Withdraws needle smoothly
- Applies pressure if indicated

Post-administration:

- Disposes of needle safely
- Documents administration
- Monitors patient response
- Provides patient education
- Reports adverse reactions

Intravenous Therapy

Intravenous therapy provides direct access to the circulatory system, allowing for rapid drug delivery and precise dosing. However, it also carries increased risks and requires specialized knowledge and skills.

IV site assessment ensures safe administration:

- Check for signs of infiltration or phlebitis
- Assess patency by checking blood return
- Evaluate site for swelling, redness, or pain
- Ensure secure catheter placement
- Monitor for complications

Flow rate calculations ensure accurate delivery:

- Calculate mL/hr for infusion pumps
- Calculate drops/minute for gravity infusions
- Account for tubing drop factor
- Verify calculations with colleagues
- Monitor actual delivery rates

Basic flow rate formula: Flow rate (mL/hr) = Total volume (mL) ÷ Time (hours)

Gravity flow formula: gtts/min = (Volume × Drop factor) ÷ (Time in minutes)

Complications and interventions:

- **Infiltration:** Fluid leaks into surrounding tissue
- **Phlebitis:** Vein inflammation
- **Infection:** Bacterial contamination
- **Air embolism:** Air bubbles in circulation
- **Fluid overload:** Excessive fluid administration

Progressive Skill: Basic to Complex IV Scenarios

Build IV therapy skills progressively:

Level 1: Basic IV assessment

- Identify normal IV site appearance
- Recognize signs of complications
- Practice documentation of IV status
- Demonstrate proper hand hygiene

Level 2: IV medication preparation

- Calculate simple IV medication doses
- Practice aseptic technique
- Demonstrate proper mixing procedures
- Show correct labeling techniques

Level 3: IV pump operation

- Program infusion pumps correctly
- Respond to pump alarms
- Calculate flow rates accurately
- Demonstrate troubleshooting skills

Level 4: Complex IV therapy

- Manage multiple IV infusions
- Calculate compatibility issues
- Handle emergency situations
- Coordinate with other therapies

Topical and Inhalation Routes

Topical and inhalation routes provide localized drug delivery with reduced systemic effects. Understanding proper application techniques ensures effectiveness and safety.

Transdermal patches deliver medications through skin:

- Remove old patch before applying new one
- Rotate application sites

- Don't cut patches
- Dispose of used patches safely
- Monitor for skin irritation

Eye medications require special techniques:

- Pull lower eyelid down to create pocket
- Don't touch dropper to eye
- Apply gentle pressure to inner corner
- Use separate bottles for each eye if infected
- Wait 5 minutes between different eye medications

Ear medications need proper positioning:

- Warm medication to room temperature
- Pull ear up and back for adults
- Pull ear down and back for children
- Don't insert dropper deeply into ear
- Keep patient positioned for 2-3 minutes

Metered-dose inhalers deliver medications to lungs:

- Shake inhaler before use
- Exhale completely before inhaling
- Form tight seal around mouthpiece
- Inhale slowly and deeply while pressing canister
- Hold breath for 10 seconds
- Rinse mouth after steroid inhalers

Hands-on Stations: Route-Specific Administration Practice

Practice specialized administration techniques:

Station 1: Transdermal patch application

- Practice site selection and rotation
- Demonstrate proper removal technique
- Show correct application procedures
- Practice disposal methods

113

Station 2: Eye drop administration

- Practice proper positioning
- Demonstrate technique for drops and ointments
- Show correct eyelid manipulation
- Practice preventing contamination

Station 3: Ear drop administration

- Practice age-appropriate ear positioning
- Demonstrate proper instillation technique
- Show correct patient positioning
- Practice documentation

Station 4: Inhaler instruction

- Practice patient education techniques
- Demonstrate proper inhaler use
- Show spacer device usage
- Practice troubleshooting common problems

Medication Safety and Error Prevention

Medication Reconciliation

Medication reconciliation is a formal process of comparing a patient's medication orders to all medications the patient has been taking. This process helps identify discrepancies and prevent errors.

Admission, transfer, discharge processes each require reconciliation:

- **Admission:** Compare home medications to admission orders
- **Transfer:** Compare current medications to transfer orders
- **Discharge:** Compare discharge medications to current regimen

Common discrepancies include:

- Medications omitted from orders
- Incorrect doses or frequencies
- Duplicate medications
- Inappropriate drug interactions
- Allergic reactions to prescribed medications

Practical Exercise: Complete Medication Reconciliation Forms

Practice reconciliation with realistic scenarios:

Scenario: Mrs. Johnson is admitted with chest pain. Her home medications include:

- Lisinopril 10 mg daily
- Metformin 500 mg twice daily
- Aspirin 81 mg daily
- Vitamin D 1000 units daily

Admission orders include:

- Lisinopril 5 mg daily
- Metformin 500 mg twice daily
- Aspirin 325 mg daily
- Atorvastatin 20 mg daily

Discrepancies identified:

- Lisinopril dose changed from 10 mg to 5 mg
- Aspirin dose increased from 81 mg to 325 mg
- Vitamin D not ordered
- Atorvastatin added

Actions required:

- Clarify reason for Lisinopril dose change
- Verify aspirin dose increase is intentional
- Determine if Vitamin D should be continued
- Ensure patient understands new medication

Patient Education

Patient education about medications is essential for safety, effectiveness, and adherence. Patients who understand their medications are more likely to take them correctly and report problems.

Teaching principles for effective education:

- Assess patient's current knowledge
- Use language appropriate for education level
- Provide written information to supplement verbal teaching
- Include family members when appropriate
- Verify understanding through teach-back method

Adherence strategies improve medication compliance:

- Simplify medication regimens when possible
- Use pill organizers for complex regimens
- Provide clear instructions about timing
- Discuss importance of completing full courses
- Address cost concerns and access issues

Cultural considerations affect medication education:

- Language barriers may require interpreters
- Cultural beliefs about medications vary
- Family involvement in healthcare decisions
- Religious considerations for certain medications
- Traditional healing practices may interact with medications

Role-Play: Patient Teaching Scenarios

Practice patient education in realistic situations:

Scenario 1: Diabetic patient starting insulin

- **Patient:** 55-year-old man newly diagnosed with diabetes

- **Medication:** Insulin glargine 20 units daily
- **Teaching needs:** Injection technique, storage, hypoglycemia recognition
- **Barriers:** Fear of needles, cost concerns

Scenario 2: Elderly patient with multiple medications

- **Patient:** 78-year-old woman with heart failure
- **Medications:** Multiple daily medications
- **Teaching needs:** Organization, timing, side effects
- **Barriers:** Memory issues, complex regimen

Scenario 3: Pediatric patient with asthma

- **Patient:** 8-year-old child with asthma
- **Medication:** Albuterol inhaler
- **Teaching needs:** Proper inhaler technique, when to use
- **Barriers:** Age-appropriate instruction, school administration

Scenario 4: Postoperative patient with pain medication

- **Patient:** 45-year-old woman after surgery
- **Medication:** Oxycodone for pain
- **Teaching needs:** Pain assessment, addiction concerns, side effects
- **Barriers:** Pain affecting concentration, family concerns

Each scenario should include:

- Assessment of learning needs
- Appropriate teaching methods
- Verification of understanding
- Plans for follow-up
- Documentation of education provided

Chapter 5 Skills Assessment

Your medication administration competency will be evaluated through comprehensive assessments:

Medication Administration OSCE

You'll demonstrate competency in:

- Rights of medication administration
- Proper calculation techniques
- Safe preparation procedures
- Correct administration techniques
- Appropriate documentation
- Patient education skills

Dosage Calculation Exam

Your mathematical competency will be assessed through:

- Basic conversion problems
- Simple dosage calculations
- Complex IV calculations
- Pediatric dosing problems
- Critical care calculations
- Real-world scenarios

Medication Error Analysis

You'll analyze medication errors to:

- Identify contributing factors
- Develop prevention strategies
- Understand system failures
- Recognize human factors
- Propose quality improvements
- Learn from others' experiences

Competency Portfolio: All Routes Demonstration

You'll compile evidence of competency in:

- Oral medication administration
- Injectable medication techniques
- IV therapy management
- Topical medication application
- Inhalation therapy instruction
- Patient education documentation

Embracing the Responsibility

Medication administration is both a privilege and a responsibility. Every time you give a medication, you're participating in a healing process that can dramatically improve someone's quality of life. The knowledge and skills you develop in this area will serve you throughout your nursing career and directly impact patient outcomes.

Remember that becoming proficient in medication administration is a continuous process. Stay current with new medications, maintain your calculation skills, and always prioritize patient safety over speed or convenience. When in doubt, ask questions, double-check calculations, and never hesitate to seek help from experienced colleagues.

The systematic approach to medication administration you've learned—from understanding pharmacology to calculating dosages to educating patients—provides a framework for safe practice. Use this framework consistently, and you'll develop the confidence and competence needed to administer medications safely in any healthcare setting.

In the next chapter, we'll explore mobility and positioning—essential skills for maintaining patient comfort, preventing complications, and promoting healing. The attention to detail and systematic approach you've developed with medication administration will serve you well in all aspects of patient care.

Key Takeaways

1. **Pharmacology knowledge enhances medication safety.** Understanding how medications work helps you anticipate effects and recognize problems.
2. **Accurate dosage calculations prevent medication errors.** Multiple calculation methods provide flexibility and verification opportunities.
3. **Route-specific techniques ensure medication effectiveness.** Each administration route requires specific knowledge and skills.
4. **Pediatric dosing requires special considerations.** Weight-based and BSA calculations help ensure safe pediatric medication administration.
5. **IV therapy carries increased risks and responsibilities.** Proper assessment and monitoring prevent serious complications.
6. **Patient education promotes safety and adherence.** Understanding medications helps patients participate effectively in their care.
7. **Medication reconciliation prevents errors during transitions.** Systematic comparison of medication lists identifies discrepancies.
8. **System-based approaches prevent medication errors.** The rights of medication administration provide a framework for safe practice.

Chapter 6: Mobility and Positioning

Watch a physical therapist help a stroke patient take their first steps after weeks of bed rest. See the determination in the patient's eyes, the gentle encouragement of the therapist, and the family members holding their breath in anticipation. This moment represents more than just walking—it represents independence, hope, and the beginning of recovery. As a nurse, you'll be part of countless moments like these, helping patients maintain and regain their mobility.

Human beings are designed to move. Our bodies function best when we're active, when our muscles contract and relax, when our joints move through their full range of motion, and when our circulatory system is challenged by changes in position. Yet illness, injury, and hospitalization often limit mobility, sometimes dramatically. When patients can't move normally, complications develop quickly: muscles weaken, joints stiffen, circulation slows, and the risk of blood clots and pressure injuries increases.

The human cost of immobility is staggering. Muscle strength can decrease by 10-15% per week of bed rest, and bone density can drop by 1% per week (27). Patients who lose mobility often struggle to regain it, leading to prolonged recovery times, increased healthcare costs, and reduced quality of life. Yet many of these complications are preventable through proper positioning, regular movement, and systematic mobility programs.

Mobility Assessment

Functional Mobility Scale

Assessing a patient's mobility helps you understand their current abilities, identify risks, and plan appropriate interventions. Functional mobility assessment goes beyond simply asking "Can you walk?" It involves systematic evaluation of various movement activities and the assistance required for each.

Common assessment tools provide standardized ways to evaluate mobility:

Barthel Index measures independence in activities of daily living:

- Feeding (0-10 points)
- Bathing (0-5 points)
- Grooming (0-5 points)
- Dressing (0-10 points)
- Bowel control (0-10 points)
- Bladder control (0-10 points)
- Toilet use (0-10 points)
- Transfers (0-15 points)
- Mobility (0-15 points)
- Stairs (0-10 points)

Functional Independence Measure (FIM) assesses 18 items in six areas:

- Self-care activities
- Sphincter control
- Transfers
- Locomotion
- Communication
- Social cognition

Timed Up and Go (TUG) test measures mobility and fall risk:

- Patient sits in chair
- Stands up without using arms
- Walks 3 meters
- Turns around
- Walks back to chair
- Sits down

Scoring:

- Less than 10 seconds: Normal
- 10-20 seconds: Good mobility

- 20-30 seconds: Mobility problems
- More than 30 seconds: Severe mobility impairment

Gait analysis basics help identify mobility problems:

- **Stance phase:** Foot is in contact with ground (60% of gait cycle)
- **Swing phase:** Foot is off the ground (40% of gait cycle)
- **Stride length:** Distance between heel strikes of same foot
- **Step length:** Distance between heel strikes of different feet
- **Cadence:** Number of steps per minute

Balance evaluation assesses fall risk:

- **Static balance:** Ability to maintain position while stationary
- **Dynamic balance:** Ability to maintain balance during movement
- **Reactive balance:** Ability to recover from perturbations

Practical Exercise: Mobility Assessment Practice

Practice systematic mobility assessment with classmates:

Assessment protocol:

1. **Observation:** Watch patient at rest and during movement
2. **Range of motion:** Assess joint flexibility and strength
3. **Transfers:** Evaluate bed-to-chair movement
4. **Ambulation:** Assess walking ability and safety
5. **Balance:** Test static and dynamic balance
6. **Endurance:** Note fatigue during activities

Documentation should include:

- Current mobility level
- Assistive devices used
- Amount of assistance required
- Safety concerns identified
- Patient goals and preferences

- Barriers to mobility

Practice scenarios:

- Post-surgical patient with pain
- Elderly patient with weakness
- Stroke patient with hemiparesis
- Patient with orthopedic injury
- Patient with chronic illness

Risk Factors for Impaired Mobility

Understanding factors that affect mobility helps you identify patients at risk and implement preventive measures. Some risk factors are modifiable, while others require adaptation of care approaches.

Age-related changes affect mobility in predictable ways:

- **Muscle mass:** Decreases by 3-8% per decade after age 30
- **Bone density:** Decreases, especially in postmenopausal women
- **Joint flexibility:** Reduces due to cartilage changes
- **Balance:** Deteriorates due to sensory and neurological changes
- **Cardiovascular fitness:** Decreases without regular exercise

Medical conditions that commonly affect mobility:

- **Neurological disorders:** Stroke, Parkinson's disease, multiple sclerosis
- **Musculoskeletal conditions:** Arthritis, fractures, amputations
- **Cardiovascular disease:** Heart failure, peripheral artery disease
- **Respiratory disease:** COPD, pulmonary fibrosis
- **Metabolic disorders:** Diabetes, thyroid dysfunction

Psychosocial factors influence mobility and recovery:

- **Fear of falling:** Can lead to activity avoidance

124

- **Depression:** Reduces motivation for activity
- **Cognitive impairment:** Affects safety awareness
- **Social isolation:** Reduces opportunities for movement
- **Cultural beliefs:** May influence activity participation

Environmental barriers limit mobility:

- **Physical obstacles:** Stairs, narrow doorways, uneven surfaces
- **Inadequate lighting:** Increases fall risk
- **Lack of assistive devices:** Limits independence
- **Institutional policies:** May restrict movement unnecessarily
- **Staffing limitations:** May reduce assistance availability

Case Study: Post-Stroke Mobility Challenges

Meet Robert Martinez, a 58-year-old man who suffered a stroke three days ago. His case illustrates the complex factors that affect mobility after a neurological event.

Medical history:

- Hypertension
- Type 2 diabetes
- Previous myocardial infarction
- Sedentary lifestyle

Current condition:

- Left-sided weakness (hemiparesis)
- Mild speech difficulties
- Blood pressure controlled with medication
- Blood glucose levels stable

Mobility assessment findings:

- **Strength:** Right side normal, left side 3/5
- **Range of motion:** Limited on left side
- **Balance:** Impaired, requires support
- **Transfers:** Requires moderate assistance

- **Ambulation:** Unable to walk independently

Risk factors identified:

- **Medical:** Stroke affects left brain hemisphere
- **Physical:** Weakness, balance problems
- **Psychological:** Frustration with limitations
- **Social:** Wife anxious about caring for him
- **Environmental:** Two-story home, bathroom upstairs

Nursing interventions:

1. **Positioning:** Prevent contractures and pressure injuries
2. **Range of motion:** Maintain joint flexibility
3. **Progressive mobility:** Gradual increase in activity
4. **Safety measures:** Fall prevention strategies
5. **Patient education:** Teach compensation techniques
6. **Family support:** Involve wife in care planning

Interdisciplinary collaboration:

- **Physical therapy:** Gait training and strengthening
- **Occupational therapy:** ADL retraining
- **Speech therapy:** Communication improvement
- **Social work:** Discharge planning and resources
- **Dietitian:** Nutrition support for recovery

Goals and outcomes:

- **Short-term:** Safe transfers with minimal assistance
- **Medium-term:** Ambulation with assistive device
- **Long-term:** Maximum independence at home
- **Family goal:** Confidence in providing care

This case demonstrates how multiple factors interact to affect mobility and how comprehensive assessment guides intervention planning.

Body Mechanics and Ergonomics

Principles of Safe Movement

Proper body mechanics protect both patients and healthcare workers from injury. Understanding these principles and applying them consistently can prevent musculoskeletal injuries that affect millions of healthcare workers annually.

Center of gravity is the point where body weight is evenly distributed:

- Located at about the level of the pelvis
- Lowers with squatting or bending
- Staying within base of support improves stability
- Moving center of gravity requires energy

Base of support is the area within the outline of body parts touching the ground:

- Wider base provides more stability
- Feet shoulder-width apart creates good base
- Moving base of support in direction of movement improves balance
- Narrower base allows for easier movement

Proper lifting technique prevents back injury:

1. **Plan the lift:** Assess weight and get help if needed
2. **Position feet:** Shoulder-width apart, close to object
3. **Squat down:** Keep back straight, bend knees
4. **Secure grip:** Use both hands, keep object close
5. **Lift smoothly:** Use leg muscles, avoid twisting
6. **Move feet:** Don't twist spine while carrying

Line of gravity is an imaginary vertical line through the center of gravity:

- Should pass through base of support for stability
- Moving outside base of support causes loss of balance
- Proper alignment keeps line of gravity centered
- Changes in position require adjustment

Activity: Body Mechanics Demonstration and Practice

Practice proper body mechanics in healthcare scenarios:

Station 1: Lifting from floor

- Demonstrate proper squatting technique
- Show incorrect lifting with bent back
- Practice with objects of different weights
- Discuss when to get help

Station 2: Moving objects laterally

- Show proper pivoting technique
- Demonstrate keeping object close to body
- Practice moving items on different surfaces
- Discuss use of sliding aids

Station 3: Reaching and bending

- Demonstrate safe reaching limits
- Show proper bending technique
- Practice retrieving objects from different heights
- Discuss use of step stools and reaching aids

Station 4: Carrying and transporting

- Show proper carrying positions
- Demonstrate use of carts and equipment
- Practice team lifting techniques
- Discuss load distribution

Key principles reinforced:

- Keep back straight and neutral
- Use large muscle groups
- Maintain good balance
- Avoid twisting motions
- Get help when needed

Healthcare Worker Safety

Healthcare workers have injury rates higher than those in construction and manufacturing (28). Understanding ergonomic principles and using available resources can significantly reduce injury risk.

Injury prevention strategies address multiple risk factors:

- **Education:** Learn proper techniques and risks
- **Fitness:** Maintain physical conditioning
- **Equipment:** Use available assistive devices
- **Environment:** Modify workspace when possible
- **Policies:** Follow safe patient handling protocols

Common injuries among healthcare workers:

- **Back injuries:** Most common, often from lifting
- **Shoulder injuries:** From reaching and lifting
- **Neck injuries:** From sustained awkward positions
- **Knee injuries:** From prolonged standing or kneeling
- **Wrist injuries:** From repetitive motions

Ergonomic risk factors in healthcare:

- **Force:** Amount of physical exertion required
- **Repetition:** Frequency of similar motions
- **Awkward postures:** Positions that stress joints
- **Duration:** Length of time in position
- **Vibration:** Tool or equipment vibration

Prevention strategies:

- **Job rotation:** Vary tasks to reduce repetition

- **Micro-breaks:** Short rest periods during tasks
- **Proper workstation setup:** Adjust height and position
- **Team lifting:** Use multiple people for heavy loads
- **Mechanical aids:** Use lifts and transfer devices

Self-Assessment: Personal Body Mechanics Evaluation

Evaluate your own body mechanics practices:

Lifting assessment:

- Do you plan lifts before beginning?
- Do you maintain proper foot position?
- Do you keep your back straight?
- Do you use leg muscles for power?
- Do you avoid twisting while lifting?

Daily activities assessment:

- Do you maintain good posture while sitting?
- Do you take breaks from prolonged positions?
- Do you use proper reaching techniques?
- Do you wear appropriate footwear?
- Do you stay physically fit?

Work environment assessment:

- Is your workspace set up ergonomically?
- Do you have access to assistive devices?
- Are you aware of safe lifting policies?
- Do you know how to report injuries?
- Are you comfortable asking for help?

Improvement plan:

- Identify areas needing improvement
- Set specific goals for change
- Practice new techniques regularly
- Seek education on proper techniques

- Monitor progress over time

Patient Positioning

Therapeutic Positions

Proper positioning is essential for patient comfort, prevention of complications, and promotion of healing. Different positions serve different therapeutic purposes and require specific techniques to ensure safety and effectiveness.

Fowler's position elevates the head of the bed:

- **High Fowler's:** 60-90 degrees, promotes breathing
- **Semi-Fowler's:** 30-45 degrees, general comfort
- **Low Fowler's:** 15-30 degrees, slight elevation
- **Uses:** Respiratory problems, feeding, comfort

Supine position places patient flat on back:

- **Standard supine:** Flat, arms at sides
- **Modifications:** Pillow under knees for comfort
- **Uses:** Procedures, examinations, rest
- **Risks:** Pressure on sacrum, heels

Prone position places patient on abdomen:

- **Standard prone:** Face down, head to side
- **Modifications:** Pillows under chest and pelvis
- **Uses:** Respiratory therapy, pressure relief
- **Risks:** Breathing difficulty, pressure on face

Lateral position places patient on side:

- **Right lateral:** On right side
- **Left lateral:** On left side
- **Modifications:** Pillows between legs
- **Uses:** Comfort, pressure relief, procedures

Trendelenburg position lowers head below feet:

- **Uses:** Shock, certain procedures
- **Risks:** Increased intracranial pressure
- **Contraindications:** Head injury, respiratory problems

Reverse Trendelenburg raises head above feet:

- **Uses:** Reduce intracranial pressure
- **Benefits:** Improved breathing
- **Considerations:** Monitor for hypotension

Position changes and frequency prevent complications:

- **Frequency:** Every 2 hours for immobile patients
- **Documentation:** Record position changes
- **Assessment:** Check skin integrity with each turn
- **Individualization:** Adjust based on patient needs

Skill Stations: Practice All Positions with Rationales

Practice positioning techniques with proper rationales:

Station 1: Fowler's positioning

- Practice adjusting bed to different angles
- Show proper pillow placement
- Demonstrate pressure point assessment
- Discuss indications for each angle

Station 2: Lateral positioning

- Practice proper body alignment
- Show pillow placement between legs
- Demonstrate support for top arm
- Discuss pressure point protection

Station 3: Prone positioning

- Practice safe turning technique
- Show proper pillow placement
- Demonstrate airway management
- Discuss contraindications

Station 4: Specialty positions

- Practice Trendelenburg positioning
- Show proper patient preparation
- Demonstrate monitoring techniques
- Discuss safety considerations

Learning objectives:

- Understand therapeutic purposes of each position
- Master safe positioning techniques
- Recognize contraindications
- Identify comfort measures
- Plan position change schedules

Pressure Injury Prevention

Pressure injuries (formerly called pressure ulcers or bed sores) are localized damage to skin and underlying tissue caused by prolonged pressure. They're largely preventable through proper positioning, skin care, and risk assessment.

Risk assessment tools help identify high-risk patients:

Braden Scale assesses six risk factors:

- **Sensory perception:** Ability to feel pressure
- **Moisture:** Degree of skin moisture
- **Activity:** Level of physical activity
- **Mobility:** Ability to change position
- **Nutrition:** Usual food intake pattern
- **Friction and shear:** Ability to move without assistance

Scoring:

- **19-23 points:** No risk
- **15-18 points:** Low risk
- **13-14 points:** Moderate risk
- **10-12 points:** High risk
- **9 or below:** Very high risk

Norton Scale evaluates five factors:

- Physical condition
- Mental state
- Activity
- Mobility
- Incontinence

Positioning devices and supports reduce pressure:

- **Pillows:** Soft, moldable pressure redistribution
- **Foam wedges:** Maintain specific angles
- **Heel protectors:** Prevent heel pressure injuries
- **Pressure-redistributing mattresses:** Specialized surfaces
- **Cushions:** For wheelchair users

Skin inspection techniques identify problems early:

- **Frequency:** With each position change
- **Areas to assess:** Bony prominences, pressure points
- **Signs to watch for:** Redness, warmth, swelling, breakdown
- **Documentation:** Record findings and interventions

Progressive Case: Developing Comprehensive Prevention Plan

Follow Mrs. Chen, an 82-year-old woman with multiple risk factors for pressure injuries:

Initial assessment:

- **Braden Score:** 12 (high risk)
- **Risk factors:** Advanced age, poor nutrition, incontinence, limited mobility

- **Skin condition:** Thin, fragile, dry
- **Current pressure points:** Sacrum, heels, elbows

Prevention plan development:

1. **Positioning schedule:** Turn every 2 hours
2. **Pressure redistribution:** Specialized mattress
3. **Skin care:** Moisture barrier cream
4. **Nutrition:** Protein supplements
5. **Activity:** Physical therapy consultation

Implementation:

- **Week 1:** Establish turning schedule, apply heel protectors
- **Week 2:** Add pressure-redistributing mattress
- **Week 3:** Increase protein intake, begin gentle exercises
- **Week 4:** Evaluate effectiveness, adjust plan

Monitoring and adjustment:

- **Daily:** Skin inspection with position changes
- **Weekly:** Reassess Braden score
- **Ongoing:** Modify plan based on skin condition
- **Documentation:** Record all assessments and interventions

Outcomes:

- **Skin integrity:** Maintained throughout hospitalization
- **Comfort:** Patient reports improved comfort
- **Family satisfaction:** Understands prevention importance
- **Cost savings:** Avoided expensive pressure injury treatment

This case demonstrates how systematic assessment and intervention prevent pressure injuries in high-risk patients.

Assistive Devices and Ambulation

Walking Aids

Walking aids help patients maintain mobility and independence while providing stability and reducing fall risk. Understanding proper fitting and instruction techniques ensures safe and effective use.

Canes provide stability and support:

- **Standard cane:** Single tip, provides minimal support
- **Quad cane:** Four-tip base, provides more stability
- **Proper height:** Top of cane at wrist level when arm hangs naturally
- **Proper technique:** Hold in hand opposite to weak side

Walkers provide maximum stability:

- **Standard walker:** Must be lifted with each step
- **Wheeled walker:** Easier to maneuver, less stable
- **Proper height:** Handles at wrist level when standing upright
- **Proper technique:** Step into walker, don't walk behind it

Crutches allow mobility with lower extremity injuries:

- **Axillary crutches:** Most common, require upper body strength
- **Forearm crutches:** More comfortable for long-term use
- **Proper fit:** 2-3 finger widths between axilla and crutch top
- **Weight bearing:** On hands, not axilla

Proper fitting ensures safety and effectiveness:

- **Height adjustment:** Patient standing upright
- **Weight distribution:** Evenly balanced
- **Grip comfort:** Handles at proper height
- **Stability:** Device doesn't wobble or shift

Gait patterns depend on weight-bearing status:

- **Three-point gait:** Non-weight-bearing on affected side
- **Four-point gait:** Partial weight-bearing both legs
- **Two-point gait:** Weight-bearing both legs

- **Swing-through gait:** For bilateral leg weakness

Hands-on Practice: Gait Training with Devices

Practice assistive device instruction and gait training:

Station 1: Cane instruction

- Practice proper fitting techniques
- Demonstrate correct hand position
- Show proper gait pattern
- Practice stair negotiation

Station 2: Walker instruction

- Practice height adjustment
- Demonstrate safe walking technique
- Show proper turning methods
- Practice sitting and standing

Station 3: Crutch instruction

- Practice proper fitting
- Demonstrate weight distribution
- Show different gait patterns
- Practice obstacle navigation

Station 4: Safety assessment

- Evaluate patient readiness
- Assess home environment needs
- Identify safety concerns
- Plan progressive training

Key teaching points:

- Proper device fit is essential
- Safety comes before speed

- Practice in safe environment first
- Regular maintenance is important
- Know when to ask for help

Transfer Equipment

Transfer equipment helps move patients safely while reducing injury risk for both patients and healthcare workers. Understanding proper use and selection criteria ensures safe patient handling.

Slide boards facilitate lateral transfers:

- **Uses:** Bed to stretcher, wheelchair to bed
- **Technique:** Bridge gap between surfaces
- **Safety:** Secure both surfaces, adequate staffing
- **Maintenance:** Clean between uses

Mechanical lifts provide safe lifting:

- **Hydraulic lifts:** Manual pump operation
- **Electric lifts:** Battery-powered operation
- **Ceiling lifts:** Mounted overhead track system
- **Portable lifts:** Mobile, battery-powered

Transfer belts provide secure grip:

- **Gait belts:** Used for ambulation assistance
- **Transfer belts:** Wider, more padding
- **Proper placement:** Around waist, not chest
- **Grip:** Underhand, close to patient

Standing aids assist with transfers:

- **Transfer boards:** Slide across surfaces
- **Pivot discs:** Reduce rotational forces
- **Transfer chairs:** Specialized seating
- **Mechanical stands:** Powered standing assistance

Simulation: Safe Transfer Scenarios

Practice transfer techniques in realistic scenarios:

Scenario 1: Bed to wheelchair transfer

- **Patient:** Post-operative, partial weight-bearing
- **Equipment:** Transfer belt, wheelchair
- **Staffing:** One nurse, patient assists
- **Technique:** Pivot transfer with belt

Scenario 2: Stretcher to bed transfer

- **Patient:** Unconscious, total care
- **Equipment:** Slide board, adequate staffing
- **Staffing:** Three people minimum
- **Technique:** Lateral transfer using board

Scenario 3: Chair to bed using mechanical lift

- **Patient:** Confused, non-weight-bearing
- **Equipment:** Mechanical lift, proper sling
- **Staffing:** Two people for safety
- **Technique:** Proper sling placement, smooth lifting

Scenario 4: Bathroom transfer

- **Patient:** Elderly, unsteady gait
- **Equipment:** Transfer belt, grab bars
- **Staffing:** One nurse, close supervision
- **Technique:** Careful positioning, privacy maintenance

Safety considerations:

- Always assess patient's ability to assist
- Use appropriate equipment for situation
- Ensure adequate staffing
- Maintain patient dignity

- Document transfer method and response

Chapter 6 Skills Assessment

Your mobility and positioning competency will be evaluated through multiple assessment methods:

Patient Positioning Competency

You'll demonstrate ability to:

- Assess positioning needs
- Position patients safely in various positions
- Use appropriate supportive devices
- Prevent pressure injuries
- Maintain patient comfort and dignity
- Document positioning interventions

Transfer Technique Evaluation

Your transfer skills will be assessed for:

- Proper body mechanics
- Appropriate equipment use
- Patient safety measures
- Effective communication
- Efficient technique
- Complication prevention

Assistive Device Teaching Demonstration

You'll show competency in:

- Proper device fitting
- Safe instruction techniques
- Gait pattern teaching
- Safety assessment
- Home preparation

- Follow-up planning

OSCE Station: Mobility and Safety Scenario

You'll manage a complex scenario involving:

- Mobility assessment
- Risk factor identification
- Appropriate intervention selection
- Safe implementation
- Patient and family education
- Interdisciplinary coordination

Restoring Movement, Restoring Hope

Mobility represents more than just physical function—it represents independence, dignity, and hope for the future. When you help a patient take their first steps after surgery, reposition someone to prevent pressure injuries, or teach a family member how to use a walker safely, you're doing more than providing physical care. You're helping restore confidence, prevent complications, and improve quality of life.

The principles and techniques you've learned in this chapter will serve you throughout your nursing career. Whether you're working with premature infants learning to move their tiny limbs, adults recovering from injuries, or elderly patients maintaining their independence, these skills will help you provide safe, effective care.

Remember that mobility is a use-it-or-lose-it proposition. Every day that a patient remains immobile, they lose strength, flexibility, and function. Your role is to help patients maintain and regain mobility whenever possible, while always prioritizing safety. The systematic approach to mobility assessment, positioning, and assistance you've learned provides a framework for making these decisions confidently.

In the next chapter, we'll explore hygiene and comfort care— fundamental aspects of nursing that directly impact patient dignity, healing, and satisfaction. The attention to patient safety and systematic approach you've developed with mobility will serve you well in all aspects of patient care.

Key Takeaways

1. **Mobility assessment guides intervention planning.** Systematic evaluation helps identify risks and appropriate interventions.
2. **Proper body mechanics prevent injuries.** Both patients and healthcare workers benefit from correct lifting and moving techniques.
3. **Positioning prevents complications.** Regular position changes and proper alignment prevent pressure injuries and other problems.
4. **Assistive devices promote independence.** Proper fitting and instruction help patients maintain mobility safely.
5. **Transfer equipment reduces injury risk.** Mechanical aids protect both patients and healthcare workers during movement.
6. **Pressure injury prevention requires systematic approach.** Risk assessment, positioning, and skin care work together to prevent complications.
7. **Patient education promotes safety.** Teaching patients and families about mobility helps prevent injuries and complications.
8. **Interdisciplinary collaboration optimizes outcomes.** Physical therapists, occupational therapists, and other professionals contribute to mobility goals.

Chapter 7: Vital Signs and Basic Assessment

You hold a thermometer in your hand, and in that simple moment, you possess one of nursing's most powerful diagnostic tools. This small device can tell you if your patient's body is fighting an infection, responding to medication, or maintaining the delicate balance that keeps us alive. But here's what makes the difference between a good nurse and a great one: understanding not just how to take a temperature, but what that number means for the person lying in the bed before you.

Vital signs aren't just numbers on a chart—they're your patient's story told in degrees, beats, and breaths. Every measurement you take provides a glimpse into what's happening inside the human body, and your ability to interpret these signs can literally mean the difference between catching a problem early and missing a medical emergency.

The beauty of vital signs lies in their simplicity and their power. With basic tools and careful technique, you can gather information that guides every aspect of patient care. But don't let this simplicity fool you. Behind each measurement lies a complex understanding of human physiology, normal variations, and the subtle changes that signal trouble ahead.

Vital Signs Overview

Think of vital signs as your patient's vital statistics—the essential measurements that tell you how well their body is functioning. We call them the "Big 5" because they form the foundation of every patient assessment: temperature, pulse, respiration, blood pressure, and pain. Some facilities include pulse oximetry as a sixth sign, recognizing its importance in modern healthcare.

Temperature reflects your body's ability to maintain thermal balance. Normal adult temperature ranges from 97.0°F to 99.5°F (36.1°C to 37.5°C), but this varies based on the measurement site, time of day, and individual factors. A fever signals infection or inflammation, while hypothermia suggests exposure, shock, or metabolic problems (29).

Pulse measures heart rate and rhythm, revealing how well the cardiovascular system is working. Normal adult pulse ranges from 60 to 100 beats per minute, but athletes may have lower resting rates, and anxiety or illness can drive rates higher. The pulse also tells you about rhythm regularity and strength of contractions.

Respiration indicates how well the lungs are oxygenating the blood and removing carbon dioxide. Normal adult respiratory rate ranges from 12 to 20 breaths per minute. Changes in rate, depth, or pattern can signal respiratory problems, pain, anxiety, or metabolic imbalances.

Blood pressure measures the force of blood against arterial walls during heart contractions and relaxation. Normal blood pressure is less than 120/80 mmHg, with elevated readings indicating cardiovascular strain or disease. Hypotension can signal dehydration, bleeding, or shock (30).

Pain is increasingly recognized as the fifth sign because of its impact on healing, mobility, and quality of life. Unlike other measurements, pain is subjective—only the patient can truly describe their experience. Pain assessment requires specific tools and techniques to quantify what can't be measured with instruments.

Pulse oximetry measures oxygen saturation in the blood, providing immediate feedback about respiratory function. Normal oxygen saturation ranges from 95% to 100% in healthy adults, though patients with chronic lung disease may have lower baseline levels.

Measurement Techniques

Accurate measurement requires proper technique, appropriate equipment, and understanding of factors that can affect readings. Small errors in technique can lead to significantly incorrect values, potentially affecting patient care decisions.

Temperature measurement varies by site and method. Oral temperatures work well for cooperative adults who haven't eaten, drunk, or smoked recently. Place the thermometer under the tongue, ensuring contact with sublingual tissue. Digital thermometers typically require 30-60 seconds for accurate readings.

Tympanic (ear) thermometers provide quick readings but require proper technique. Pull the ear canal straight—up and back for adults, down and back for children under three. Insert the probe gently and press the button. Remember that ear wax or recent ear surgery can affect accuracy.

Temporal artery thermometers scan across the forehead, following the temporal artery. Start at the center of the forehead and slide across to the hairline. Some models require scanning behind the ear if the patient is diaphoretic. These thermometers work well for children and unconscious patients.

Pulse measurement requires finding the right location and using proper technique. The radial pulse at the wrist is most common for routine assessment. Place two fingertips (never your thumb) over the radial artery, just below the wrist crease on the thumb side. Apply gentle pressure until you feel the pulsation.

Count the pulse for a full 60 seconds if you detect irregularities. For regular pulses, counting for 30 seconds and multiplying by two provides adequate accuracy. Note not just the rate, but also the rhythm (regular or irregular) and quality (strong, weak, or thready).

Other pulse points include the carotid (neck), brachial (inner arm), femoral (groin), popliteal (behind knee), and dorsalis pedis (top of foot). Each serves specific purposes—carotid for CPR, brachial for blood pressure measurement, and peripheral pulses for circulation assessment.

Respiratory assessment requires observation and counting without the patient's awareness, as conscious breathing often changes patterns. Watch chest rise and fall while appearing to take the pulse. Count for

30 seconds and multiply by two for regular breathing, or count for a full minute if you notice irregularities.

Observe breathing depth (shallow, normal, or deep), rhythm (regular or irregular), and effort (easy or labored). Note any use of accessory muscles, nasal flaring, or abnormal sounds. Position affects breathing—sitting upright usually provides the most accurate assessment.

Blood pressure measurement requires proper cuff size, positioning, and technique. The cuff width should be 40% of the arm circumference, and the cuff should encircle 80% of the arm. Too small a cuff gives falsely high readings; too large gives falsely low readings.

Position the patient with their arm at heart level, feet flat on the floor, and back supported. Place the cuff snugly around the bare upper arm, with the bladder centered over the brachial artery. The bottom edge should be one inch above the elbow crease.

For manual measurement, place the stethoscope bell over the brachial artery. Inflate the cuff rapidly to 20-30 mmHg above the estimated systolic pressure. Deflate slowly at 2-3 mmHg per second while listening for Korotkoff sounds. The first sound indicates systolic pressure; the disappearance of sounds indicates diastolic pressure.

Pain assessment uses various scales and approaches. The numeric rating scale (0-10) works well for most adults. Ask patients to rate their pain from 0 (no pain) to 10 (worst possible pain). For patients who struggle with numbers, consider the faces pain scale or descriptive words (none, mild, moderate, severe).

Use the PQRST method for comprehensive pain assessment. Ask what provokes or relieves the pain (P), the quality or character of the pain (Q), the region and radiation pattern (R), the severity on a scale (S), and the timing or pattern (T). This systematic approach ensures you gather complete information about the pain experience.

Basic Physical Assessment

A systematic approach to physical assessment helps you gather information efficiently while building rapport with your patient. Think of it as detective work—you're looking for clues about your patient's condition while making them feel comfortable and respected.

Mental status assessment begins the moment you enter the room. Is your patient alert and responsive? Do they know who they are, where they are, and what day it is? Orientation to person, place, and time provides basic information about neurological function.

Observe your patient's general appearance. Do they look their stated age? Are they well-groomed or disheveled? Do they appear comfortable or distressed? These observations provide clues about their overall condition and ability to care for themselves.

Skin assessment reveals important information about circulation, hydration, and overall health. Normal skin appears pink (in lighter skin tones) or consistent with baseline coloring (in darker skin tones), feels warm and dry, and springs back quickly when gently pinched (good turgor).

Look for changes in color—pallor may indicate anemia or poor circulation, cyanosis suggests inadequate oxygenation, and jaundice can signal liver problems. Feel the skin for temperature (warm, cool, or hot) and moisture (dry, moist, or diaphoretic). Check turgor by gently pinching skin on the back of the hand or sternum; slow return suggests dehydration.

Cardiovascular assessment starts with observing for signs of adequate circulation. Are the fingers and toes warm and pink? Can you feel pulses in the feet? Are there signs of swelling (edema) in the legs or feet?

Listen to heart sounds at four main areas: aortic (second intercostal space, right sternal border), pulmonic (second intercostal space, left sternal border), tricuspid (fourth intercostal space, left sternal border), and mitral (fifth intercostal space, left midclavicular line). Normal heart sounds include S1 ("lub") and S2 ("dub"). Additional sounds like S3 or S4 may indicate heart problems.

Respiratory assessment involves both observation and auscultation. Watch for signs of respiratory distress: rapid breathing, use of accessory muscles, pursed-lip breathing, or cyanosis around the lips or fingernails.

Listen to lung sounds in a systematic pattern, comparing side to side. Normal breath sounds are clear and equal bilaterally. Abnormal sounds include crackles (fine, moist sounds suggesting fluid), wheezes (musical sounds suggesting airway narrowing), and rhonchi (coarse, wet sounds suggesting secretions).

Abdominal assessment follows a specific sequence: inspection, auscultation, percussion, and palpation. Look for distension, asymmetry, or visible pulsations. Listen for bowel sounds in all four quadrants—normal sounds occur every 5-15 seconds and have a gurgling quality.

Gentle palpation can detect tenderness, masses, or organ enlargement. Start with light palpation in areas away from any reported pain, then progress to deeper palpation if appropriate. Remember that abdominal assessment requires advanced training, so focus on basic observation and reporting abnormal findings.

Recording and Reporting

Accurate documentation protects your patients, your colleagues, and yourself. Every vital sign measurement and assessment finding should be recorded promptly and accurately, with attention to both the numbers and any relevant observations.

Documentation standards require specific information for each vital sign. Record the actual measurement, the method used (oral thermometer, right radial pulse), and any relevant factors (patient was anxious, just returned from physical therapy). Include the date, time, and your signature or initials according to facility policy.

Use proper abbreviations and terminology. Temperature is recorded as degrees Fahrenheit or Celsius with the route noted (T 98.6°F PO for oral temperature). Pulse includes rate and rhythm (P 88 regular). Respirations note rate and character (R 16 regular and unlabored). Blood pressure includes both systolic and diastolic pressures with patient position (BP 120/80 sitting).

When to report abnormal findings depends on your patient's condition and facility protocols. Generally, you should immediately report temperatures over 101°F (38.3°C) or below 96°F (35.5°C), pulse rates over 100 or under 60 beats per minute, respiratory rates over 24 or under 10 breaths per minute, and blood pressure over 140/90 or systolic pressure under 90 mmHg.

Pain scores of 7 or higher typically require immediate attention, as do sudden changes in pain character or location. Oxygen saturation below 95% in most patients warrants prompt evaluation and intervention.

Consider the whole picture when deciding what to report. A pulse of 110 might be normal for a patient with a fever but concerning for someone at rest. A blood pressure of 100/60 might be normal for a young, healthy adult but problematic for an elderly patient taking blood pressure medications.

Electronic documentation requires careful attention to accuracy and timeliness. Most systems allow real-time entry, which helps ensure accuracy and prevents forgotten entries. Use dropdown menus and templates when available, but don't let them replace critical thinking about your patient's condition.

Practical Exercise

Let's practice with a realistic scenario. Mrs. Johnson is a 68-year-old woman admitted yesterday for pneumonia. It's 2:00 PM, and you're assigned to take her vital signs and do a basic assessment.

You enter the room and find Mrs. Johnson sitting up in bed, looking slightly flushed. She greets you appropriately and knows she's in the hospital for pneumonia. Her skin feels warm and slightly moist, and you notice she's breathing a bit faster than normal.

Vital signs measurements:

- Temperature: 100.8°F (oral)
- Pulse: 96 beats per minute, regular, strong
- Respirations: 24 per minute, slightly labored
- Blood pressure: 138/84 mmHg
- Pain: 3/10, described as chest tightness with deep breathing
- Oxygen saturation: 94% on 2 liters oxygen via nasal cannula

Documentation example: "2:00 PM - Vital signs: T 100.8°F PO, P 96 regular and strong, R 24 slightly labored, BP 138/84 sitting, Pain 3/10 chest tightness with deep inspiration, O2 sat 94% on 2L NC. Patient alert and oriented x3, skin warm and moist, respirations slightly increased from baseline. Lungs with fine crackles in bilateral lower lobes. Patient reports feeling 'a little warm' but otherwise comfortable. Dr. Smith notified of elevated temperature and increased respiratory rate. - J. Nurse, RN"

This documentation includes all measured values, relevant observations, patient statements, and actions taken. The narrative provides context that helps other healthcare providers understand the patient's condition.

Case Study: Mr. Rodriguez's Concerning Change

Mr. Rodriguez, a 45-year-old construction worker, was admitted three days ago for surgery to repair a hernia. He's been recovering well, but during your 6:00 AM vital signs check, you notice some changes that concern you.

His temperature is 101.2°F (compared to 98.4°F yesterday), his pulse is 110 beats per minute (up from his usual 75), and his blood pressure is 95/60 mmHg (down from his normal 125/80). He rates his pain as 8/10, significantly higher than the 3/10 he reported yesterday. He appears restless and says he feels "really awful" and nauseated.

Your assessment reveals that his surgical site looks more red and swollen than yesterday, with a small amount of yellowish drainage. His skin feels hot and dry, and he says he's been having chills. These findings suggest a possible surgical site infection with developing sepsis.

You immediately notify the surgeon and prepare to obtain blood cultures and start IV antibiotics as ordered. You increase the frequency of vital sign monitoring and begin documenting the patient's response to treatment. This scenario demonstrates how vital signs changes can signal serious complications requiring immediate intervention.

Case Study: Mrs. Chen's Blood Pressure Dilemma

Mrs. Chen, an 82-year-old woman with a history of hypertension, is admitted for heart failure management. Her blood pressure medications were adjusted yesterday, and you're monitoring her response. During your morning assessment, her blood pressure is 88/50 mmHg, significantly lower than her usual readings in the 140s/80s range.

She reports feeling dizzy when she sits up and says her vision gets "spotty" when she stands. Her pulse is 58 beats per minute (down from her usual 70s), and she appears pale and tired. These findings suggest that her blood pressure medications may be too strong for her current condition.

You help her remain lying flat and notify her physician about the hypotension and symptoms. The doctor orders holding her morning blood pressure medications and obtaining an electrocardiogram to check for heart rhythm changes. You continue frequent blood pressure monitoring and ensure Mrs. Chen remains safe by keeping her bed low and the call bell within reach.

This case illustrates how vital signs monitoring helps assess medication effectiveness and detect adverse effects that require prompt intervention.

Case Study: Tommy's Fever Investigation

Tommy is a 6-year-old boy brought to the emergency department by his parents because he's been feverish and cranky for two days. His oral temperature is 103.2°F, pulse is 130 beats per minute, respirations are 28 per minute, and blood pressure is 90/55 mmHg. His pain score is difficult to assess because he's crying, but he points to his ear when asked what hurts.

His parents report he's been pulling at his right ear and hasn't been eating well. Your assessment reveals a red, bulging right eardrum and tender lymph nodes in his neck. His skin is hot and flushed, and he's mildly dehydrated based on decreased skin turgor and dry mucous membranes.

These findings are consistent with acute otitis media (ear infection). You prepare for antibiotic treatment and focus on comfort measures including fever reduction and pain management. You educate the parents about medication administration and signs that would require immediate return to the hospital.

This pediatric case demonstrates how vital signs interpretation differs in children and how assessment findings help establish diagnosis and guide treatment plans.

Building Assessment Skills

Developing competent assessment skills takes practice and patience. Start with healthy volunteers to learn normal findings, then gradually work with patients under supervision. Each patient teaches you something new about the variations in normal findings and the subtle signs that indicate problems.

Practice your technique until measurements become automatic. The more comfortable you become with the mechanics of taking vital signs, the more attention you can pay to interpreting what they mean for your patient's condition.

Learn to see patterns rather than isolated measurements. A single elevated blood pressure reading might mean nothing, but a trend of increasing pressures over several hours tells a different story. Context matters as much as the numbers themselves.

Trust your instincts when something doesn't seem right. New nurses often dismiss their concerns, thinking they lack experience. But your fresh eyes and careful attention to detail can catch changes that others might miss. Always report concerns to experienced nurses or physicians—they can help you determine if your observations are significant.

Bringing It All Together

Vital signs and basic assessment form the foundation of nursing practice. These skills connect you directly to your patient's physiology and provide the information needed to make clinical decisions. The temperature that signals infection, the blood pressure that reveals medication effectiveness, the pain score that guides comfort measures—each measurement contributes to the larger picture of patient care.

Excellence in these fundamental skills builds confidence and competence that serves you throughout your nursing career. The systematic approach you develop now will adapt to specialty areas and advanced practice, but the core principles remain constant: accuracy, attention to detail, and understanding of what the findings mean for patient care.

Your ability to gather, interpret, and act on assessment data makes you an essential member of the healthcare team. These skills represent the bridge between nursing science and nursing art—the technical competence and caring presence that define excellent nursing practice.

Building Clinical Confidence

Mastering these essential skills opens the door to more advanced nursing practice. Each accurate measurement builds your confidence, and each correct interpretation strengthens your clinical judgment. The patience you take to learn proper technique now pays dividends in the critical moments when your skills can make the difference in patient outcomes.

Key Learning Points

- **Master proper technique for each measurement** to ensure accuracy and reliability of your findings
- **Understand normal ranges and variations** based on age, condition, and individual factors
- **Recognize patterns and trends** rather than focusing only on isolated measurements
- **Document findings completely and accurately** including measurements, observations, and actions taken
- **Report abnormal findings promptly** based on established protocols and clinical judgment
- **Use systematic approaches** to ensure thorough and consistent patient assessment
- **Practice regularly** to build confidence and maintain competency in these fundamental skills

Chapter 8: Nutrition and Hydration

The evening meal tray sits untouched on Mrs. Patterson's bedside table. For the third day in a row, she's eaten less than half of her food, and her family asks you with worried faces why she won't eat. You understand their concern—food represents comfort, care, and healing in our minds. But you also know that helping Mrs. Patterson improve her nutrition requires understanding the complex factors that affect appetite, swallowing, and digestion in illness.

Nutrition in healthcare settings is rarely as simple as placing food in front of someone and expecting them to eat. Pain medications reduce appetite. Surgery affects digestion. Illness changes taste. Positioning matters for swallowing safety. The foods that once brought pleasure may now seem unappealing or even threatening.

Your role in supporting nutrition goes far beyond delivering meal trays. You become a detective, figuring out why patients aren't eating. You become a problem-solver, finding ways to make nutrition appealing and safe. You become an advocate, ensuring that nutritional needs don't get overlooked in the focus on medical treatments.

Basic Nutrition Principles

Think of nutrition as fuel for healing. Just as a car needs the right type and amount of gasoline to run properly, the human body needs specific nutrients to repair tissues, fight infection, and maintain strength. The three macronutrients—protein, carbohydrates, and fats—each serve distinct functions in recovery and health maintenance.

Protein acts as the building blocks for tissue repair and immune function. Patients recovering from surgery, fighting infections, or healing wounds need more protein than healthy individuals. Good sources include lean meats, fish, eggs, dairy products, beans, and nuts. The body can't store protein like it stores fat, so patients need adequate daily intake to support healing processes (31).

Carbohydrates provide immediate energy for cellular functions and brain activity. Complex carbohydrates from whole grains, fruits, and vegetables offer sustained energy and important vitamins. Simple carbohydrates from sugars provide quick energy but little nutritional value. For patients with diabetes, carbohydrate timing and amount become critical factors in blood sugar management.

Fats support vitamin absorption, hormone production, and provide concentrated energy. While patients often view fats negatively, healthy fats from sources like olive oil, avocados, and fish play important roles in recovery. Some vitamins (A, D, E, and K) require fat for absorption, making adequate fat intake necessary for proper nutrition.

Special diets address specific medical conditions and treatment requirements. Clear liquid diets provide hydration and minimal residue for patients with gastrointestinal problems or before certain procedures. Full liquid diets add nutrition while maintaining easy digestion for patients with swallowing difficulties or after certain surgeries.

Low-sodium diets help manage fluid retention in patients with heart failure, kidney disease, or hypertension. Diabetic diets focus on consistent carbohydrate intake and timing to maintain stable blood sugar levels. Renal diets restrict protein, sodium, potassium, and phosphorus for patients with kidney disease.

Texture-modified diets address swallowing difficulties through pureed foods, thickened liquids, or mechanically soft textures. These modifications maintain nutrition while reducing aspiration risk for patients with dysphagia or other swallowing disorders.

Assisting with Feeding

Safe feeding requires understanding both the mechanics of swallowing and the individual needs of each patient. Positioning, timing, food texture, and environmental factors all influence feeding success and safety.

Proper positioning is essential for safe swallowing. Patients should sit upright at 90 degrees or as close to upright as possible. This position uses gravity to help food move down the esophagus and reduces the risk of aspiration into the lungs. Patients who can't sit fully upright should be positioned at least 45 degrees with their head slightly flexed forward.

Support the patient's posture with pillows as needed. Feet should be flat on the floor or footrests, and arms should be supported. Comfortable positioning helps patients focus on eating rather than maintaining balance or managing discomfort.

Feeding techniques vary based on the patient's abilities and needs. For patients who can feed themselves, your role involves ensuring they have appropriate utensils, opening packages, cutting food into manageable pieces, and providing encouragement. Some patients need adaptive equipment like built-up handles, weighted utensils, or plate guards to eat independently.

For patients requiring feeding assistance, maintain their dignity by explaining what you're doing and following their preferred pace. Offer small bites and allow adequate time for chewing and swallowing. Sit at eye level when possible, making the experience more social and less clinical.

Recognizing swallowing difficulties protects patients from serious complications. Signs of dysphagia include coughing or choking during eating, a wet or gurgly voice after swallowing, food pocketing in the cheeks, and complaints that food "gets stuck." Patients may also avoid certain textures, eat very slowly, or refuse foods they previously enjoyed.

Aspiration precautions reduce the risk of food or liquid entering the lungs. These include maintaining upright positioning, offering small amounts, ensuring the patient is fully alert before feeding, and having suction equipment readily available. Some patients require thickened liquids to slow the swallowing process and reduce aspiration risk.

Never rush feeding or force food into a patient's mouth. If a patient shows signs of choking or distress, stop feeding immediately and assess their condition. Call for help if the patient cannot clear their airway or shows signs of respiratory distress.

Intake and Output Monitoring

Fluid balance affects every body system, from kidney function to blood pressure to mental status. Accurate intake and output (I&O) monitoring helps healthcare providers assess hydration status, kidney function, and response to treatments like diuretics or IV therapy.

Understanding fluid needs helps you recognize when patients may be at risk for dehydration or fluid overload. Healthy adults need approximately 30-35 mL of fluid per kilogram of body weight daily, though this varies based on activity level, climate, and health status. Illness often increases fluid needs through fever, increased respiratory rate, or fluid losses from vomiting or diarrhea.

Measuring intake includes all fluids entering the body—oral fluids, IV medications, tube feeding, and irrigation solutions. Common measurements include 8 ounces (240 mL) for a standard cup, 4 ounces (120 mL) for a juice glass, and 6 ounces (180 mL) for a coffee cup. Ice chips count as approximately half their volume when melted.

Keep measurement tools handy—graduated cylinders for measuring remaining fluids, conversion charts for common containers, and calculators for fluid calculations. Record intake promptly to avoid forgetting amounts or making estimation errors.

Measuring output includes all fluids leaving the body—urine, stool, vomitus, drainage from tubes, and wound drainage. Use graduated cylinders or collection containers with measurement markings for accuracy. Empty collection devices at regular intervals to prevent overflow and maintain accuracy.

Urine output should average 30 mL per hour or 0.5 mL per kilogram per hour for adequate kidney function. Less than this amount (oliguria) may indicate dehydration, kidney problems, or medication effects. Excessive urine output (polyuria) can result from diabetes, medications, or fluid overload.

Documentation standards require recording intake and output amounts, times, and characteristics. Note the color, consistency, and any unusual characteristics of output. Include running totals for each shift and 24-hour periods to help healthcare providers assess trends and make treatment decisions.

Hydration and IV Basics

Intravenous therapy provides direct access to the bloodstream for fluid replacement, medication administration, and nutritional support. Understanding basic IV care helps you recognize complications and maintain safe therapy.

Signs of dehydration include decreased skin turgor, dry mucous membranes, concentrated urine, decreased urine output, increased heart rate, and decreased blood pressure. Mental status changes like confusion or irritability may occur in severe dehydration. Elderly patients and those with chronic illnesses are particularly vulnerable to dehydration complications.

Signs of fluid overload include swelling (edema) in the legs, hands, or face, shortness of breath, rapid weight gain, and elevated blood pressure. Patients may report feeling "puffy" or that their rings or shoes are tight. Lung sounds may reveal crackles indicating fluid in the alveoli.

IV site assessment should occur at least every shift and whenever you access the IV line. Look for signs of infiltration (IV fluid leaking into surrounding tissue), phlebitis (vein inflammation), and infection. Normal IV sites appear pink, feel cool to slightly warm, and show no swelling or drainage.

Infiltration signs include swelling, coolness, and pallor around the IV site. The patient may report pain or pressure at the site. Severe infiltration can cause tissue damage, especially with certain medications. Stop the IV immediately if you suspect infiltration and notify the healthcare provider.

Phlebitis signs include redness, warmth, swelling, and a palpable cord along the vein. The patient typically reports pain or tenderness at the site. Phlebitis can progress to serious complications including blood clots, so immediate intervention is necessary.

Infection signs include redness, swelling, warmth, drainage, and streaking up the arm from the IV site. The patient may have fever or feel generally unwell. IV-related infections can become serious quickly, requiring immediate medical attention and usually IV removal.

Enteral Nutrition

Feeding tubes provide nutrition for patients who cannot eat safely by mouth but have functioning gastrointestinal systems. Understanding basic tube feeding principles helps you provide safe care and recognize complications.

Types of feeding tubes serve different purposes and durations. Nasogastric (NG) tubes go through the nose to the stomach and work well for short-term feeding. Percutaneous endoscopic gastrostomy (PEG) tubes go directly through the abdominal wall to the stomach for long-term nutrition needs.

Jejunostomy tubes go to the small intestine and may be used for patients at high risk for aspiration or those with stomach problems. Each type requires specific care techniques and has different complication risks.

Tube placement verification ensures safe feeding and medication administration. Never assume a tube is in the correct position—verify placement before each feeding or medication administration. Methods include checking pH of gastric aspirate, measuring external tube length, and obtaining X-ray confirmation when indicated.

Feeding administration requires attention to formula type, rate, and patient tolerance. Elevate the head of the bed to at least 30 degrees during feeding and for one hour afterward to reduce aspiration risk. Start feedings slowly and advance gradually as tolerated to prevent gastrointestinal upset.

Monitor for signs of intolerance including nausea, vomiting, diarrhea, cramping, or high gastric residuals. High residuals (more than 250-500 mL depending on facility protocol) may indicate delayed gastric emptying or feeding intolerance.

Tube maintenance involves keeping the feeding tube patent and the insertion site clean. Flush tubes with water before and after feedings and medications to prevent clogging. Clean around the insertion site daily and monitor for signs of irritation or infection.

Case Study: Mrs. Anderson's Post-Surgical Nutrition Challenge

Mrs. Anderson, a 72-year-old retired teacher, underwent bowel surgery five days ago to remove a section of intestine affected by diverticulitis. Her surgery went well, but she's struggling with eating and maintaining adequate nutrition during her recovery.

Current situation: Mrs. Anderson has been allowed clear liquids for two days and advanced to full liquids yesterday. However, she's only consuming about 25% of what's offered. She complains that everything tastes "awful" and that eating makes her nauseated. Her daughter reports that Mrs. Anderson was always a good eater before surgery and loved cooking for her family.

Assessment findings: Mrs. Anderson appears tired and has lost 8 pounds since admission. Her mouth is dry, and her skin turgor is slightly delayed, suggesting mild dehydration. She rates her surgical pain as 4/10, which she says is manageable. Her bowel sounds are present but sluggish, and she hasn't had a bowel movement since surgery.

Contributing factors to poor intake:

- Pain medications affecting appetite and causing nausea
- Altered taste sensation common after anesthesia and surgery
- Limited food options with liquid diet restrictions
- Anxiety about eating causing discomfort or complications
- Unfamiliar hospital environment affecting comfort with eating
- Disrupted normal eating patterns and preferences

Nursing interventions:

1. **Collaborate with the dietary team** to identify liquid options that appeal to Mrs. Anderson. Offer familiar flavors and foods she enjoyed before surgery.
2. **Coordinate pain medication timing** with meals to reduce nausea while maintaining adequate pain control. Consider anti-nausea medication before meals.
3. **Provide mouth care** before meals to improve taste and reduce the metallic taste some patients experience after surgery.
4. **Create a pleasant eating environment** by reducing noise, removing unpleasant odors, and positioning Mrs. Anderson comfortably.
5. **Offer frequent small amounts** rather than large portions that may seem overwhelming.
6. **Include family in meal planning** by asking about Mrs. Anderson's food preferences and involving her daughter in encouraging eating.

Progress and outcomes: After implementing these interventions, Mrs. Anderson's intake gradually improved. The anti-nausea medication helped significantly, and she found that chicken broth and vanilla ice cream were more palatable than other options. By day seven, she was tolerating soft solids and expressing interest in food again. Her weight stabilized, and her energy level began improving.

Case Study: Mr. Johnson's Swallowing Difficulties

Mr. Johnson, a 68-year-old man, suffered a stroke six days ago that affected his ability to speak clearly and swallow safely. The speech-language pathologist completed a swallowing evaluation and recommended a pureed diet with thickened liquids to reduce his aspiration risk.

Current challenges: Mr. Johnson becomes frustrated during meals because the pureed food doesn't look like "real food" to him. He tries to refuse meals or attempts to drink regular liquids when staff aren't watching. His wife is distressed seeing him struggle and wants to help but doesn't understand the swallowing precautions.

Safety concerns: Mr. Johnson coughed several times during his last meal and had a wet-sounding voice afterward, suggesting possible aspiration. He's at high risk for pneumonia if he continues to aspirate food or liquid into his lungs.

Nursing interventions:

1. **Educate Mr. Johnson and his wife** about dysphagia and aspiration risks using simple language and visual aids.
2. **Ensure proper positioning** for all meals—upright at 90 degrees with slight forward head flexion.
3. **Create appetizing pureed meals** by working with dietary staff to mold pureed foods into recognizable shapes and add appropriate seasonings.
4. **Supervise all oral intake** to ensure Mr. Johnson follows swallowing precautions and doesn't attempt thin liquids.
5. **Use cueing techniques** to remind Mr. Johnson to take small bites, chew thoroughly, and swallow completely before taking another bite.
6. **Involve his wife in meal assistance** after teaching her proper feeding techniques and safety precautions.

Outcomes: With consistent implementation of swallowing precautions and family education, Mr. Johnson's intake improved while maintaining safety. His wife became comfortable helping with meals, and the dietary team created more appealing pureed options. Follow-up swallowing evaluations showed gradual improvement, and Mr. Johnson was eventually able to progress to mechanically soft foods.

Case Study: Sarah's Diabetes Management Challenge

Sarah is a 16-year-old high school student with Type 1 diabetes who was admitted for diabetic ketoacidosis after missing several insulin doses. She's now medically stable but struggling with meal planning and carbohydrate counting during her hospitalization.

Presenting issues: Sarah admits she often skips meals to avoid giving insulin injections at school. She says carbohydrate counting is "too complicated" and that she just guesses most of the time. Her blood sugar levels have been erratic, ranging from 60 to 350 mg/dL over the past 24 hours.

Educational needs: Sarah needs intensive education about the relationship between food, insulin, and blood sugar control. She also needs practical strategies for managing diabetes during her busy teenage lifestyle.

Nursing interventions:

1. **Assess Sarah's current knowledge** about diabetes management and identify specific learning needs.
2. **Provide hands-on carbohydrate counting practice** using real foods and restaurant menu items that appeal to teenagers.
3. **Discuss practical strategies** for managing diabetes at school, including talking to school nurses and planning for sports activities.
4. **Involve the diabetes educator** for specialized teaching about insulin adjustment and continuous glucose monitoring options.
5. **Address psychological aspects** of diabetes management, including body image concerns and peer pressure related to food choices.
6. **Connect Sarah with other teenagers** who successfully manage diabetes for peer support and practical tips.

Long-term planning: Sarah worked with the healthcare team to develop a realistic diabetes management plan that fits her lifestyle. She learned to use a smartphone app for carbohydrate counting and arranged for backup insulin supplies at school. Follow-up appointments were scheduled to monitor her progress and adjust her management plan as needed.

Practical Applications

Supporting patient nutrition requires flexibility, creativity, and persistence. Every patient brings unique challenges—cultural food preferences, physical limitations, medication effects, and personal beliefs about food and eating. Your success depends on understanding these individual factors and adapting your approach accordingly.

Develop relationships with dietary staff, speech-language pathologists, and other team members who contribute to nutrition care. These collaborative relationships help you access resources and expertise that benefit your patients.

Stay current with evidence-based nutrition practices and your facility's policies regarding feeding assistance, tube feeding, and nutritional supplements. Nutrition science continues advancing, and new approaches may offer better outcomes for your patients.

Nourishing Recovery

Nutrition and hydration form the foundation for healing and recovery. Your attention to these basic needs can significantly impact patient outcomes and satisfaction. The patient who maintains adequate nutrition recovers faster, has fewer complications, and feels more capable of participating in their care.

Beyond the physiological benefits, food represents comfort, culture, and caring. The time you spend helping a patient eat, the effort you make to find foods they enjoy, and the attention you pay to their hydration needs communicate that you care about their overall well-being, not just their medical condition.

Key Learning Points

- **Understand the role of macronutrients** in healing and recovery for all patient populations
- **Master safe feeding techniques** including proper positioning and aspiration precautions
- **Accurately monitor intake and output** to assess hydration status and treatment effectiveness
- **Recognize signs of fluid imbalance** and understand when to report concerning findings
- **Provide safe enteral nutrition care** including tube placement verification and complication recognition
- **Adapt nutrition support** to individual patient needs, preferences, and cultural considerations
- **Collaborate with interdisciplinary team members** to optimize nutrition outcomes for all patients

Chapter 9: Elimination

The conversation every nursing student dreads—talking about toileting, bowel movements, and bladder function with patients. Yet here's the truth: elimination is as essential to health as breathing and eating. Your comfort with these topics and your skill in providing elimination care directly affects your patients' comfort, dignity, and recovery.

Elimination problems touch every aspect of a person's life. The businessman who can't control his bladder after prostate surgery. The elderly woman too weak to reach the bathroom safely. The teenager with a new colostomy struggling with body image. Each faces not just physical challenges, but emotional ones that require your understanding and support.

Your role extends far beyond emptying bedpans and changing adult briefs. You become a guardian of dignity, ensuring privacy and respect during vulnerable moments. You become an educator, teaching patients about normal elimination patterns and ways to maintain continence. You become an advocate, ensuring that elimination needs don't get ignored in busy healthcare environments.

Supporting Toileting Needs

Toileting is one of our most private activities, yet illness often makes it a public concern. The independence we take for granted— recognizing the urge, reaching a toilet, and controlling our muscles— can be compromised by surgery, medications, weakness, or cognitive changes.

Maintaining dignity during toileting assistance requires attention to privacy, communication, and respect. Always explain what you plan to do and ask permission before proceeding. Use appropriate draping to maintain modesty, close doors and curtains, and limit the number of people present to those necessary for safety.

Timing matters for successful toileting. Many patients develop predictable patterns—needing to void shortly after waking, having bowel movements after meals, or requiring assistance every two hours. Learning these patterns helps you anticipate needs and prevents accidents that embarrass patients and create extra work.

Scheduled toileting works well for patients with cognitive impairment or those learning to regain continence. Offer toileting opportunities every two hours during waking hours, after meals, and before bedtime. Even if patients don't express the need, regular opportunities often prevent accidents and maintain normal elimination patterns.

Environmental modifications support independence and safety. Ensure clear pathways to the bathroom, adequate lighting, and accessible call systems. Remove scatter rugs, provide nonslip footwear, and consider raised toilet seats or grab bars for patients with mobility limitations.

Bedpan and urinal use requires proper technique to ensure comfort and safety. Warm metal bedpans before use to increase comfort. Position patients properly—semi-Fowler's position for bedpans, standing or sitting for urinals when possible. Provide privacy by leaving the room when safe to do so, or at least avoiding direct eye contact during use.

Urinary Care

The urinary system eliminates waste products and maintains fluid balance, making proper urinary function critical for overall health. Understanding normal urination patterns helps you recognize problems and provide appropriate interventions.

Normal urination patterns vary among individuals but follow general guidelines. Healthy adults typically void 4-8 times during a 24-hour period, producing 1500-3000 mL of urine daily. Urine should be pale yellow, clear, and have a mild odor. Changes in frequency, amount, color, or odor may signal problems requiring investigation.

Catheter care basics focus on maintaining sterile technique and preventing complications. Indwelling urinary catheters (Foley catheters) require specific care techniques to reduce infection risk and maintain proper function.

Perineal hygiene becomes especially important for catheterized patients. Clean the urethral opening and surrounding area with soap and water daily and after bowel movements. Clean from front to back for female patients to prevent bacterial contamination from the anal area.

Drainage bag management requires attention to positioning and emptying procedures. Keep drainage bags below bladder level at all times to prevent urine backflow and potential infection. Secure bags to prevent pulling on the catheter, which can cause trauma and discomfort.

Empty drainage bags when they're two-thirds full or at least every 8 hours using sterile technique. Use separate measuring containers for each patient to prevent cross-contamination. Record output amounts and note urine characteristics including color, clarity, and odor.

Catheter security prevents accidental removal and reduces trauma. Secure catheters to the thigh for female patients and to the abdomen or thigh for male patients using appropriate securing devices. Ensure enough slack to prevent tension during movement while maintaining proper drainage bag position.

Promoting Urinary Health

Prevention remains the best approach to maintaining urinary health and preventing complications. Understanding risk factors and implementing preventive measures protects patients from serious complications like urinary tract infections and kidney problems.

Preventing urinary tract infections requires multiple strategies. Encourage adequate fluid intake (2-3 liters daily unless contraindicated) to flush bacteria from the urinary system. Promote complete bladder emptying by ensuring patients take adequate time for voiding and aren't rushed.

For catheterized patients, maintain sterile technique during catheter insertion and care. Avoid unnecessary catheter use and remove catheters as soon as medically appropriate. The risk of infection increases with catheter duration, making early removal a priority.

Recognizing urine abnormalities helps identify problems early. **Cloudy urine** may indicate infection, especially when accompanied by strong odor or burning during urination. **Dark yellow or amber urine** suggests dehydration and need for increased fluid intake.

Red or pink urine requires immediate investigation as it may indicate bleeding from anywhere in the urinary tract. However, certain foods (beets, berries) and medications can also cause red-colored urine. **Brown or tea-colored urine** may suggest liver problems or severe dehydration.

Strong, foul-smelling urine often indicates infection, while **sweet-smelling urine** may suggest diabetes. **Foamy urine** can indicate protein in the urine, which may signal kidney problems.

Encouraging regular voiding helps maintain normal bladder function and prevents complications. Teach patients not to delay urination when they feel the urge, as this can lead to incomplete emptying and increased infection risk. For hospitalized patients, offer toileting opportunities regularly rather than waiting for requests.

Bowel Care

Bowel elimination removes waste products and maintains the body's chemical balance. Normal bowel patterns vary widely among individuals, making it important to understand each patient's typical patterns rather than applying universal standards.

Normal bowel patterns range from three times daily to three times weekly, depending on diet, activity level, medications, and individual factors. Stool should be brown, formed but not hard, and passed without straining or discomfort. Changes in frequency, consistency, or characteristics may indicate problems.

Managing constipation requires understanding contributing factors and implementing appropriate interventions. Common causes include decreased activity, inadequate fluid intake, low-fiber diet, medications (especially opioids), and ignoring the urge to defecate.

Dietary interventions for constipation include increasing fiber intake through fruits, vegetables, and whole grains. Prunes contain natural substances that promote bowel movements and work well for many patients. Adequate fluid intake (2-3 liters daily unless contraindicated) helps soften stool and promote elimination.

Activity promotion stimulates bowel function through physical movement. Even bed-bound patients benefit from range-of-motion exercises and position changes. Walking and other physical activities promote normal bowel function for mobile patients.

Managing diarrhea focuses on preventing dehydration and identifying underlying causes. Encourage fluid replacement with clear liquids, and monitor for signs of dehydration including decreased skin turgor, dry mucous membranes, and decreased urine output.

Bedpan and commode use requires proper technique and attention to safety. Position patients comfortably and provide privacy. For bedbound patients, elevate the head of the bed to facilitate elimination. Ensure call bells are within reach and respond promptly to requests.

Enema administration may be necessary for constipation or bowel preparation. Types include cleansing enemas (soap suds, saline), retention enemas (oil), and medicated enemas. Always check orders carefully and follow facility protocols for administration techniques and patient monitoring.

Incontinence Care

Incontinence affects millions of people and can significantly impact quality of life, self-esteem, and social functioning. Understanding different types of incontinence and appropriate management strategies helps you provide effective, compassionate care.

Types of incontinence have different causes and treatment approaches. **Stress incontinence** occurs with coughing, sneezing, or physical activity and results from weakened pelvic floor muscles. **Urge incontinence** involves sudden, strong urges to urinate with inability to delay voiding.

Overflow incontinence occurs when the bladder doesn't empty completely, leading to frequent small voids or constant dribbling. **Functional incontinence** results from physical or cognitive barriers to reaching the toilet in time despite normal bladder function.

Skin care becomes critical for incontinent patients to prevent breakdown and infection. Change wet or soiled garments and linens promptly. Clean the skin gently with mild soap and water, and dry thoroughly. Apply barrier creams to protect skin from moisture and irritation.

Absorbent products include adult briefs, pads, and underpads designed to manage incontinence while maintaining dignity. Choose products appropriate for the amount and type of incontinence. Change products promptly when soiled to prevent skin problems and odor.

Emotional support addresses the psychological impact of incontinence. Many patients feel embarrassed, frustrated, or depressed about losing control over this basic function. Provide reassurance that incontinence is a medical condition, not a personal failure. Maintain matter-of-fact approach to care while acknowledging patients' feelings.

Bladder training programs can help some patients regain continence. These involve scheduled voiding at gradually increasing intervals to retrain the bladder to hold larger volumes. Success requires patient cooperation and consistent implementation.

Case Study: Mr. Thompson's Post-Operative Urinary Retention

Mr. Thompson, a 58-year-old accountant, underwent hernia repair surgery yesterday under spinal anesthesia. Eight hours after surgery, he hasn't urinated despite drinking plenty of fluids and feeling the urge to void. He's becoming increasingly uncomfortable and anxious about his inability to urinate.

Assessment findings: Mr. Thompson's bladder is palpable above the pubic bone, and he reports feeling "really full" but unable to start his urine stream. He's tried standing, sitting, and different positions without success. His vital signs are stable except for mild elevation in blood pressure, which he attributes to discomfort.

Contributing factors:

- Spinal anesthesia effects on bladder innervation
- Pain medications affecting bladder muscle function
- Anxiety about urinating with others nearby
- Unfamiliar hospital environment and positioning
- Possible bladder muscle dysfunction from prolonged retention

Nursing interventions:

1. **Provide privacy** by closing curtains, ensuring the room is quiet, and giving Mr. Thompson time alone to attempt voiding.
2. **Try positioning changes** including standing at the bedside if stable, or sitting on the edge of the bed with feet flat on the floor.
3. **Use relaxation techniques** such as running water, placing hands in warm water, or pouring warm water over the perineum to stimulate voiding.
4. **Monitor for bladder distension** by palpating the abdomen and measuring bladder volume with a bladder scanner if available.

5. **Collaborate with the physician** regarding possible need for catheterization if conservative measures fail.

Outcome: After trying various positioning and relaxation techniques, Mr. Thompson was able to void 600 mL of urine while standing at the bedside. His discomfort resolved immediately, and he was able to urinate normally for the remainder of his hospitalization. This case demonstrates how simple interventions can often resolve post-operative urinary retention without invasive procedures.

Case Study: Mrs. Garcia's Bowel Management Challenge

Mrs. Garcia, a 78-year-old woman with dementia, lives in a long-term care facility. Over the past week, she's had several episodes of fecal incontinence that have distressed her family and challenged the nursing staff. She's normally continent and follows a regular toileting schedule.

Recent changes: Mrs. Garcia started a new antibiotic five days ago for a urinary tract infection. She's also been eating less than usual and appears more confused than her baseline. The incontinence episodes have occurred at various times without apparent pattern.

Assessment considerations:

- Antibiotic effects on normal intestinal bacteria causing diarrhea
- Decreased oral intake affecting stool consistency
- Increased confusion affecting awareness of elimination needs
- Possible connection between UTI treatment and bowel function
- Need to differentiate between diarrhea and overflow incontinence

Nursing interventions:

1. **Review medication effects** and discuss with the physician the possibility of antibiotic-associated diarrhea.

2. **Implement more frequent toileting** schedule to accommodate changes in bowel patterns.
3. **Monitor food and fluid intake** to ensure adequate nutrition and identify any dietary triggers.
4. **Provide immediate skin care** after incontinence episodes using gentle cleansing and barrier protection.
5. **Consider probiotics** to restore normal intestinal flora disrupted by antibiotic therapy.
6. **Educate family members** about temporary nature of antibiotic-related bowel changes and expected improvement.

Resolution: Mrs. Garcia's bowel function gradually normalized as her antibiotic course ended and normal intestinal bacteria were restored. The addition of probiotics and increased attention to toileting schedule prevented further episodes. Her family felt reassured understanding the temporary medical cause of the incontinence.

Case Study: Jennifer's New Ostomy Adjustment

Jennifer, a 28-year-old nurse, underwent emergency surgery for inflammatory bowel disease that resulted in a temporary colostomy. Three days post-operatively, she's struggling emotionally with the ostomy and refusing to look at or participate in ostomy care.

Emotional challenges: Jennifer expresses shock and disgust about the ostomy, saying she "can't handle being a nurse with this thing." She's worried about returning to work, maintaining relationships, and managing the ostomy independently. She asks repeatedly about reversal surgery and seems to focus only on that possibility.

Physical challenges: The ostomy is functioning normally, producing formed stool. However, Jennifer's refusal to participate in care is limiting her learning and preparation for discharge. The ostomy site appears healthy without signs of complications.

Nursing approaches:

1. **Acknowledge Jennifer's feelings** and validate that adjusting to an ostomy is emotionally challenging for anyone, especially healthcare workers.
2. **Provide gradual exposure** by first having Jennifer touch the ostomy bag while you perform care, then progress to watching care, and finally participating in care steps.
3. **Connect with ostomy nurse specialist** for expert guidance and peer support resources.
4. **Arrange peer support** with other nurses who have ostomies and successfully returned to work.
5. **Focus on temporary nature** of the ostomy while also preparing Jennifer for all possibilities regarding reversal surgery.
6. **Address practical concerns** about working as a nurse with an ostomy, including uniform modifications and break schedules.

Long-term outcomes: With supportive counseling and gradual exposure, Jennifer became comfortable with ostomy care and returned to nursing practice six weeks later. She found that her experience as an ostomy patient made her more empathetic and effective when caring for other patients with similar challenges. The ostomy was successfully reversed six months later as planned.

Quick Skills Check

Proper bedpan assistance sequence:

1. Gather supplies (bedpan, toilet paper, washcloths, towels)
2. Explain procedure and ensure privacy
3. Raise bed to working height and lower side rail
4. Help patient lift hips or turn to side for bedpan placement
5. Position bedpan with wider end toward patient's back
6. Raise head of bed to comfortable sitting position
7. Provide call bell and leave patient alone if safe
8. Return promptly when called
9. Lower head of bed and remove bedpan carefully
10. Provide perineal care and hand hygiene
11. Empty and clean bedpan using proper infection control

12. Document elimination including amount and characteristics

Catheter drainage bag emptying procedure:

1. Perform hand hygiene and gather supplies
2. Put on clean gloves
3. Clean drainage spout with alcohol wipe
4. Open drainage spout into graduated cylinder
5. Allow bag to empty completely without touching spout to cylinder
6. Close drainage spout and clean again
7. Measure and record output
8. Empty graduated cylinder and clean
9. Remove gloves and perform hand hygiene
10. Document output amount and urine characteristics

Maintaining Human Dignity

Elimination care represents nursing at its most fundamental level—helping people with basic human needs while preserving their dignity and promoting their health. The technical skills matter, but the compassion and respect you bring to these intimate moments matter more.

Every patient facing elimination challenges—temporary or permanent—deserves care that acknowledges their humanity. The businessman with urinary retention, the woman with incontinence, the young adult with a new ostomy—each requires not just skilled care but understanding and support as they navigate these challenges.

Your comfort with elimination topics and your skill in providing this care become gifts you give to vulnerable patients. The professional, matter-of-fact way you approach these needs helps patients feel less embarrassed and more willing to ask for help when needed.

Key Learning Points

- **Understand normal elimination patterns** and recognize deviations that require intervention or physician notification
- **Master proper techniques** for bedpan use, catheter care, and incontinence management while maintaining patient dignity
- **Implement infection prevention strategies** especially for catheterized patients and those with elimination problems
- **Recognize signs of complications** including urinary tract infections, constipation, and skin breakdown from incontinence
- **Provide compassionate emotional support** for patients struggling with elimination challenges and body image changes
- **Educate patients and families** about normal elimination promotion and management strategies
- **Document elimination patterns accurately** including frequency, characteristics, and any concerning changes

Chapter 10: Medication Administration

You stand at the medication cart, double-checking the five rights one more time before entering your patient's room. The small pill in your hand represents years of research, careful prescribing, and now your final verification before it enters another human being. This moment—repeated thousands of times daily in healthcare facilities worldwide—carries enormous responsibility and potential.

Medication administration stands as one of nursing's most high-stakes activities. Done correctly, medications heal diseases, relieve suffering, and save lives. Done incorrectly, they can cause harm, disability, or death. The difference often lies not in the medication itself, but in the knowledge, attention to detail, and systematic approach of the nurse administering it.

Your role extends far beyond simply giving medications. You become the final safety check in a complex system. You become an educator, helping patients understand their treatments. You become an advocate, questioning orders that don't seem right and reporting concerns that could prevent errors.

Medication Basics

Understanding what medications do and how they work helps you anticipate effects, recognize problems, and educate patients effectively. While you don't need to memorize every drug detail, you need enough knowledge to administer medications safely and recognize when something isn't right.

Medications serve several purposes in healthcare. Some treat underlying diseases—antibiotics fight infections, antihypertensives lower blood pressure, and insulin regulates blood sugar. Others provide symptom relief—analgesics reduce pain, antiemetics prevent nausea, and bronchodilators open airways.

Your nursing role in medication administration encompasses multiple responsibilities. You verify that the right patient receives the right medication in the right dose by the right route at the right time. You assess patients before and after medication administration. You educate patients about their medications and monitor for therapeutic effects and adverse reactions.

Understanding drug actions helps you anticipate what to expect. Onset refers to how quickly a medication begins working—IV medications work within minutes, while some oral medications take hours. Duration indicates how long effects last—some medications work for hours, others for days.

Therapeutic effects are the desired actions of medications. Analgesics should reduce pain, antihypertensives should lower blood pressure, and antibiotics should clear infections. Monitor patients for these expected effects to evaluate medication effectiveness.

Side effects are undesired but expected medication effects. Many patients experience drowsiness with opioid pain medications, stomach upset with certain antibiotics, or dizziness with blood pressure medications. Understanding common side effects helps you educate patients and monitor appropriately.

Adverse reactions are unexpected or dangerous medication effects that require immediate attention. These include allergic reactions, toxic effects, or severe side effects that threaten patient safety. Recognizing and responding quickly to adverse reactions can prevent serious complications.

The Five Rights

The five rights of medication administration provide a systematic framework for safe medication practices. These rights serve as checkpoints to prevent errors and ensure patient safety throughout the medication administration process.

Right patient verification requires using two patient identifiers before every medication administration. Ask patients to state their name and date of birth, and compare this information to their identification band and medication administration record. Never rely on room numbers or bed assignments for patient identification.

Barcode scanning systems provide additional verification but don't replace your responsibility to confirm patient identity. If barcodes don't scan properly or systems are down, use manual verification methods according to facility protocols.

Right medication verification involves comparing the medication order to the actual medication multiple times. Check the medication name when removing it from storage, when preparing it for administration, and before giving it to the patient. Be especially careful with look-alike and sound-alike medications.

Pay attention to both generic and brand names, as the same medication may be known by different names. For example, acetaminophen and Tylenol are the same medication. If you're unfamiliar with a medication, look it up in a reliable reference before administering it.

Right dose calculation and verification prevents dosing errors that can cause serious harm. Calculate doses carefully using appropriate formulas and conversion factors. Double-check calculations, especially for high-alert medications or when doses seem unusually large or small.

Pay attention to decimal points, which can make ten-fold differences in doses. Question orders that require breaking tablets in unusual ways or giving large numbers of tablets or capsules. When in doubt, ask a colleague to verify your calculations.

Right route selection ensures medications reach their intended destination in the body. Oral medications must be swallowed, sublingual medications dissolve under the tongue, and topical medications are applied to the skin. Never change the route of administration without a physician's order.

Some medications are available in multiple formulations for different routes. Ensure you're using the correct formulation—IV morphine is much more concentrated than oral morphine, and using the wrong one could be fatal.

Right time administration maintains therapeutic blood levels and prevents medication interactions. Give medications within the time frames specified by facility policy—usually within 30 minutes to one hour of the scheduled time. Some medications have stricter timing requirements based on their actions.

Consider factors that affect timing, such as meals, other medications, and patient activities. Some medications must be given with food, others on an empty stomach. Some cannot be given together due to interactions.

Additional rights enhance medication safety beyond the basic five. The **right to refuse** acknowledges that competent patients can decline medications. Document refusals and notify physicians as appropriate.

Right documentation creates a legal record of medication administration. Document immediately after giving medications, including time, dose, route, and patient response. Never document medications before giving them.

Right assessment involves evaluating patients before and after medication administration. Check vital signs, pain levels, or other relevant parameters before giving medications. Monitor for therapeutic effects and adverse reactions after administration.

Routes of Administration

Different routes of medication administration offer advantages and disadvantages depending on the medication, patient condition, and desired effects. Understanding these differences helps you administer medications safely and educate patients effectively.

Oral medications are convenient, safe, and preferred for most patients. They include tablets, capsules, liquids, and sublingual preparations. Oral medications are absorbed through the gastrointestinal tract, making onset slower than other routes but effects longer-lasting.

Tablet administration requires ensuring patients can swallow safely. Position patients upright and provide adequate liquid for swallowing. Some tablets can be crushed if patients have swallowing difficulties, but many cannot—extended-release, enteric-coated, and sublingual tablets must remain intact.

Liquid medications work well for patients with swallowing difficulties or those requiring precise dosing. Measure liquids at eye level using appropriate measuring devices. Shake suspensions before measuring to ensure proper mixing.

Sublingual medications dissolve under the tongue for rapid absorption. Common examples include nitroglycerin for chest pain and some pain medications. Instruct patients not to swallow, eat, drink, or smoke until the medication dissolves completely.

Topical medications are applied to the skin for local or systemic effects. Clean the application site before applying medication. Wear gloves to protect yourself from medication absorption. Apply thin, even layers unless directed otherwise.

Transdermal patches deliver medication through the skin over extended periods. Remove old patches before applying new ones, and rotate application sites to prevent skin irritation. Fold used patches in half with the medication side inside before disposal.

Injectable medications provide rapid, predictable effects by bypassing the digestive system. Routes include intradermal (into the skin), subcutaneous (under the skin), intramuscular (into muscle), and intravenous (into bloodstream).

Subcutaneous injections work well for medications requiring slow, steady absorption. Common sites include the outer upper arms, abdomen, and thighs. Rotate injection sites to prevent tissue damage, especially important for patients taking insulin multiple times daily.

Use proper needle size—typically 25-27 gauge and 3/8 to 5/8 inch length. Insert at 45-90 degree angles depending on patient size and medication requirements. Aspiration (pulling back on the syringe) is no longer routinely recommended for subcutaneous injections.

Intramuscular injections provide faster absorption than subcutaneous routes. Common sites include the deltoid muscle in the upper arm, vastus lateralis in the thigh, and ventrogluteal area in the hip. Use proper landmarks to avoid nerves and blood vessels.

Choose appropriate needle size based on patient size and injection site—typically 20-25 gauge and 1-1.5 inches long. Use Z-track technique for medications that can irritate tissues by pulling skin to one side before insertion, then releasing after injection.

Administration Procedures

Systematic medication administration procedures reduce error risk and ensure consistent, safe practices. Following established routines helps prevent missed steps and promotes patient safety throughout the process.

Reading the MAR (Medication Administration Record) carefully starts every medication pass. Review each patient's medications, noting times, doses, routes, and any special instructions. Check for new orders, discontinued medications, and PRN (as needed) medications that patients might need.

Verifying orders ensures you're working with current, complete information. Check that orders are legible, complete, and properly signed. Question any orders that seem unclear, incomplete, or inappropriate for the patient's condition.

Preparing medications requires attention to detail and proper technique. Gather all supplies needed for each patient's medications. Work in a quiet area free from distractions. Prepare medications for one patient at a time to prevent mix-ups.

Checking calculations prevents dosing errors that can harm patients. Use appropriate formulas for dosage calculations and unit conversions. Have a colleague verify calculations for high-alert medications or when doses seem unusual.

Drawing up injections requires sterile technique and attention to accuracy. Check medication vials for cracks, expiration dates, and clarity. Use appropriate syringes and needles for each medication and route. Remove air bubbles to ensure accurate dosing.

Observing administration means staying with patients until they take oral medications completely. Don't leave medications at the bedside for patients to take later unless specifically ordered. Ensure patients actually swallow medications rather than hiding them in their mouths.

Monitoring patient response begins immediately after medication administration. Watch for signs of allergic reactions, especially with new medications. Monitor vital signs when indicated. Assess for therapeutic effects and side effects according to medication profiles.

Preventing Errors

Medication errors can occur at any step in the medication process, from prescribing to administration. Understanding common error types and prevention strategies helps you maintain patient safety and prevent harm.

System-based prevention reduces reliance on individual memory and attention. Use barcode scanning when available. Follow standard protocols for medication preparation and administration. Minimize interruptions during medication administration.

Double-checking procedures provide additional verification for high-risk medications. Two nurses should independently verify insulin doses, anticoagulant doses, and chemotherapy medications. Both nurses should sign the medication record when required.

Avoiding distractions during medication preparation and administration reduces error risk. Establish quiet zones for medication preparation. Wear distinctive vests or badges during medication administration to signal others not to interrupt. Complete medication tasks before moving to other activities.

High-alert medications require special precautions due to their potential for causing serious harm. These include insulin, anticoagulants, opioids, chemotherapy agents, and concentrated electrolytes. Use extra verification steps and monitoring for these medications.

Look-alike and sound-alike medications pose special challenges. Examples include celebrex and cerebyx, or humalog and humulin. Use both generic and brand names when communicating about medications. Store similar medications separately when possible.

Error reporting helps prevent future occurrences and improve patient safety. Report all medication errors and near-misses according to facility policies. Focus on system improvements rather than individual blame. Learn from errors to prevent similar occurrences.

Case Study: Pain Management Challenge

Mrs. Williams, a 65-year-old woman, underwent major abdominal surgery yesterday and is experiencing significant pain that's affecting her recovery. She rates her pain as 8/10 despite receiving scheduled pain medications. Her nurse must assess the situation and safely manage her pain while following medication administration principles.

Current situation: Mrs. Williams received her last dose of oxycodone 10 mg four hours ago and is eligible for another dose. She also has orders for morphine 2-4 mg IV every 2 hours as needed for breakthrough pain. She appears uncomfortable, is reluctant to move, and says the pain is preventing her from sleeping.

Assessment findings: Mrs. Williams is alert and oriented, with stable vital signs except for slightly elevated blood pressure (148/92) and heart rate (95). She has good respiratory effort with oxygen saturation of 96% on room air. Her surgical incision appears normal without signs of complications.

Medication administration considerations:

1. **Right patient:** Verify Mrs. Williams' identity using two identifiers
2. **Right medication:** Confirm morphine order and check for any allergies
3. **Right dose:** Determine appropriate dose within ordered range (2-4 mg)
4. **Right route:** Prepare for IV administration using proper technique
5. **Right time:** Ensure adequate time has passed since last opioid dose

Nursing actions:

1. **Assess pain thoroughly** using numeric scale and PQRST method to understand pain characteristics
2. **Review medication history** to check previous doses and patient response
3. **Check for contraindications** including respiratory status and level of consciousness
4. **Administer morphine 3 mg IV** after proper verification and preparation
5. **Monitor patient response** including pain relief, vital signs, and respiratory status
6. **Document administration** including dose, time, patient response, and any side effects

Follow-up care: Thirty minutes after morphine administration, Mrs. Williams reports pain decreased to 4/10. Her vital signs remain stable, and she's able to participate in deep breathing exercises. The nurse documents the positive response and continues monitoring for both therapeutic effects and potential side effects.

Case Study: Insulin Administration Safety

Mr. Garcia, a 58-year-old man with type 2 diabetes, requires insulin administration according to a sliding scale based on his blood glucose levels. His morning blood glucose is 285 mg/dL, requiring careful calculation and administration of rapid-acting insulin.

Sliding scale orders:

- Blood glucose 150-199: 2 units insulin aspart
- Blood glucose 200-249: 4 units insulin aspart
- Blood glucose 250-299: 6 units insulin aspart
- Blood glucose 300-349: 8 units insulin aspart
- Blood glucose over 350: Call physician

Calculation and verification: Based on Mr. Garcia's blood glucose of 285 mg/dL, he requires 6 units of insulin aspart according to the sliding scale. This is a high-alert medication requiring double verification with another nurse before administration.

Safety procedures implemented:

1. **Double-check calculation** with second nurse—both independently calculate required dose
2. **Verify insulin type** ensuring rapid-acting insulin aspart is used, not long-acting insulin
3. **Use insulin syringe** marked in units, not a standard syringe
4. **Check expiration date** and inspect insulin for clarity (should be clear, not cloudy)
5. **Confirm injection site** and rotate from previous injection locations

Administration technique: The nurse cleans the injection site on Mr. Garcia's abdomen, pinches the skin gently, and inserts the needle at a 90-degree angle. After injecting the insulin, the needle is removed quickly and disposed of in a sharps container. The injection site is not massaged to avoid affecting absorption.

Post-administration monitoring: The nurse monitors Mr. Garcia for signs of hypoglycemia over the next 2-4 hours, as rapid-acting insulin peaks during this time. She educates him about hypoglycemia symptoms and ensures he has access to appropriate snacks if blood sugar drops too low.

Case Study: Multiple Medication Coordination

Mr. Patterson, a 75-year-old man with heart failure, hypertension, and diabetes, takes multiple medications that require careful timing and monitoring. His morning medications include several that can interact or affect his condition.

Morning medication schedule:

- Furosemide (Lasix) 40 mg PO - diuretic for heart failure
- Lisinopril 10 mg PO - ACE inhibitor for blood pressure
- Metformin 500 mg PO - diabetes medication
- Digoxin 0.25 mg PO - heart medication
- Potassium chloride 20 mEq PO - electrolyte replacement

Assessment before administration: The nurse checks Mr. Patterson's vital signs: blood pressure 142/88, heart rate 68 and regular, respirations 18, oxygen saturation 94%. His most recent lab results show potassium 3.8 mEq/L (normal), digoxin level 1.2 ng/mL (therapeutic), and creatinine 1.4 mg/dL (slightly elevated).

Medication considerations:

1. **Furosemide** can cause potassium loss, making potassium supplementation important
2. **Lisinopril** can increase potassium levels and affect kidney function
3. **Digoxin** requires monitoring heart rate—hold if pulse below 60
4. **Metformin** should be given with food to reduce stomach upset
5. **Potassium** should be given with food and adequate fluid to prevent stomach irritation

189

Safe administration sequence: The nurse gives the medications with Mr. Patterson's breakfast to improve absorption and reduce stomach upset. She monitors his heart rate throughout and would hold digoxin if the pulse dropped below 60. She educates him about the importance of taking medications as prescribed and reporting any concerning symptoms.

Advanced Administration Considerations

PRN (as needed) medication administration requires additional assessment and decision-making skills. Before giving PRN medications, assess whether the patient actually needs them based on current symptoms and previous responses. Document not only when PRN medications are given, but also when they're offered and refused.

Medication timing around procedures may require holding or adjusting doses. Some medications need to be stopped before surgery, while others must be continued. Blood pressure medications might be held if patients are NPO (nothing by mouth), while diabetes medications require adjustment based on eating schedules.

Patient education about medications improves safety and compliance. Explain what each medication does, common side effects to expect, and serious effects to report immediately. Use simple language and provide written information when possible. Verify understanding by having patients explain key points back to you.

Cultural considerations may affect medication acceptance and compliance. Some cultures prefer herbal remedies or have religious restrictions about certain medications. Work with patients and families to find acceptable solutions that maintain medical effectiveness while respecting cultural beliefs.

Medication reconciliation at admission, transfer, and discharge prevents dangerous omissions or duplications. Compare home medications to hospital orders and clarify any discrepancies with physicians. Ensure patients understand any changes to their home medication regimens.

Technology and Medication Safety

Barcode medication administration systems reduce errors by verifying patient identity, medication, dose, and timing electronically. However, technology doesn't replace critical thinking—always verify that scanned information makes sense for the patient's condition and ordered treatments.

Automated dispensing systems improve medication security and tracking while providing decision support. These systems can alert you to drug interactions, allergies, or unusual doses. Pay attention to these alerts and investigate any concerns before proceeding.

Electronic health records provide access to patient information, medication histories, and clinical decision support. Use these tools to verify allergies, check recent lab results, and review medication effectiveness. However, always validate electronic information with direct patient assessment.

Smart pumps for IV medications provide dosing calculations and safety alerts. Program pumps carefully and respond appropriately to alarms. Understand that smart pumps are tools to assist you, not replace your clinical judgment about appropriate medication therapy.

Building Medication Competence

Developing expertise in medication administration requires continuous learning and practice. Start by mastering basic principles and gradually build knowledge about specific medication classes and complex administration techniques.

Use reliable resources for medication information, including facility formularies, drug reference books, and electronic databases. Don't rely on memory alone—look up unfamiliar medications before administering them.

Learn from experienced nurses who can share practical tips and help you recognize potential problems. Ask questions about medications you're unfamiliar with and observe experienced nurses managing complex medication regimens.

Practice calculations regularly to maintain proficiency in dosage computations. Many facilities require annual competency testing for medication calculations, but regular practice helps you maintain skills and confidence.

Stay current with new medications, changing protocols, and safety initiatives. Attend educational programs, read professional journals, and participate in facility-sponsored medication safety activities.

Safeguarding Lives Through Vigilance

Medication administration represents one of nursing's most critical responsibilities. The decisions you make, the attention you pay to detail, and the systematic approach you follow can prevent serious harm and promote healing. Each medication you give correctly contributes to patient recovery and demonstrates your commitment to safe practice.

The complexity of modern medication regimens requires nurses who understand not just the mechanical aspects of giving medications, but the physiological effects, potential interactions, and individual patient factors that influence medication safety and effectiveness. Your role as the final checkpoint in the medication process makes you an essential guardian of patient safety.

Excellence in medication administration builds confidence and competence that serves you throughout your nursing career. The habits you develop now—careful verification, thorough assessment, patient education, and systematic documentation—become the foundation for safe practice in any clinical setting.

Key Learning Points

- **Master the five rights** of medication administration and use them consistently for every medication given
- **Understand basic pharmacology** including onset, duration, therapeutic effects, and common side effects of major medication classes
- **Use proper technique** for all routes of medication administration while maintaining sterile technique when indicated
- **Implement safety measures** including double-checking high-alert medications and using available technology appropriately
- **Assess patients thoroughly** before and after medication administration to evaluate effectiveness and detect adverse reactions
- **Educate patients effectively** about their medications to promote safety and compliance
- **Document completely and accurately** all medication administration including patient responses and any concerns
- **Report errors and near-misses** to contribute to system improvements and prevent future occurrences

Chapter 11: Skin Integrity and Wound Care

The human skin spans approximately 20 square feet and weighs about 8 pounds, making it the body's largest organ. Yet most of us take this remarkable barrier for granted until something goes wrong. A surgical incision that won't heal. A pressure injury that develops during a hospital stay. A diabetic foot ulcer that threatens amputation. Suddenly, this protective covering becomes a source of pain, infection risk, and healing challenges that affect every aspect of a person's life.

Your understanding of skin integrity and wound care can mean the difference between rapid healing and prolonged complications. The elderly woman who develops a pressure injury during bed rest. The surgical patient whose incision becomes infected. The diabetic man whose small foot wound becomes a serious threat to his mobility. Each depends on your knowledge and skills to prevent problems and promote healing.

Skin and wound care represents nursing at its most fundamental level—protecting the body's first line of defense and supporting its natural healing processes. The principles you learn here apply to every patient you'll ever care for, from preventing pressure injuries in immobilized patients to managing complex surgical wounds.

Skin as the First Line of Defense

Think of skin as your body's personal armor—a sophisticated barrier that protects against infection, regulates temperature, prevents fluid loss, and provides sensory information about the environment. Understanding how healthy skin functions helps you recognize when problems develop and know how to support healing.

Normal skin structure consists of three layers, each serving specific protective functions. The epidermis forms the outermost barrier, constantly renewing itself as old cells are shed and new ones form. This layer contains no blood vessels but depends on the deeper layers for nutrition and oxygen.

The dermis contains blood vessels, nerve endings, hair follicles, and sweat glands. This layer provides skin strength and elasticity while housing the structures that regulate temperature and provide sensation. The hypodermis (subcutaneous layer) contains fat cells that provide insulation and cushioning.

Skin functions extend far beyond simple protection. The skin regulates body temperature through blood vessel dilation and constriction, plus sweating and shivering responses. It synthesizes vitamin D when exposed to sunlight and serves as a reservoir for fat and water.

Normal healing process follows predictable phases that overlap and depend on adequate nutrition, oxygenation, and protection from further injury. The inflammatory phase begins immediately after injury, bringing increased blood flow and immune cells to the area. This causes the redness, swelling, and warmth associated with early healing.

The proliferative phase follows, during which new tissue forms to fill the wound defect. Blood vessels grow into the area, and collagen fibers provide strength to the healing tissue. Finally, the maturation phase can last months to years as the new tissue strengthens and reorganizes.

Factors affecting healing include age, nutrition, circulation, medications, and underlying health conditions. Older adults heal more slowly due to decreased circulation and thinner skin. Poor nutrition deprives tissues of the protein and vitamins needed for repair. Diabetes, smoking, and certain medications can significantly impair healing (32).

Assessment techniques for skin integrity involve systematic inspection and palpation of all skin surfaces. Look for changes in color, texture, temperature, and moisture. Note any lesions, rashes, or areas of breakdown. Pay special attention to bony prominences where pressure injuries commonly develop.

Document skin findings using appropriate terminology. **Erythema** refers to redness, **edema** to swelling, and **induration** to hardness or firmness. **Maceration** describes skin softening from excessive moisture, while **excoriation** refers to surface abrasions from scratching or friction.

Pressure Injury Prevention

Pressure injuries (formerly called pressure ulcers or bedsores) represent one of healthcare's most preventable complications, yet they continue to affect millions of patients annually. Understanding risk factors and implementing evidence-based prevention strategies can eliminate most pressure injuries.

Understanding pressure injury development helps you recognize at-risk patients and implement appropriate interventions. Pressure injuries occur when sustained pressure, friction, or shear forces damage skin and underlying tissues. Areas over bony prominences are most vulnerable because tissues are compressed between bone and external surfaces.

Risk assessment tools help identify patients most likely to develop pressure injuries. The Braden Scale evaluates six factors: sensory perception, moisture, activity, mobility, nutrition, and friction/shear. Scores range from 6-23, with lower scores indicating higher risk. Scores of 18 or below typically trigger prevention protocols (33).

Braden Scale components each address specific risk factors:

- **Sensory perception** assesses ability to feel pressure and discomfort
- **Moisture** evaluates skin exposure to dampness from incontinence or sweating
- **Activity** measures degree of physical activity and time spent in bed/chair
- **Mobility** assesses ability to change and control body position
- **Nutrition** evaluates usual food intake patterns and nutritional status

- **Friction and shear** addresses problems with skin sliding against sheets or surfaces

Prevention strategies address modifiable risk factors through systematic interventions. **Repositioning schedules** should occur at least every two hours for bed-bound patients and every hour for chair-bound patients. Use pillows, foam wedges, or positioning devices to maintain proper alignment and reduce pressure on vulnerable areas.

Pressure redistribution surfaces include specialized mattresses, overlays, and cushions designed to spread pressure over larger surface areas. These range from simple foam overlays to complex alternating pressure systems. Choose surfaces based on patient risk level, comfort, and clinical effectiveness.

Skin care protocols focus on keeping skin clean and dry while maintaining natural protective barriers. Use mild, pH-balanced cleansers and avoid hot water that can damage fragile skin. Apply moisturizers to prevent dryness and cracking, but avoid over-moisturizing areas prone to maceration.

Nutrition support provides the building blocks needed for healthy skin maintenance and healing. Ensure adequate protein intake (1.2-1.5 grams per kilogram body weight for at-risk patients), calories, vitamins C and A, and zinc. Consider nutritional supplements for patients with poor oral intake.

Basic Wound Care

Wound care combines scientific principles with practical skills to support the body's natural healing processes. Understanding wound types, assessment techniques, and treatment principles prepares you to care for most wounds you'll encounter in clinical practice.

Wound classification helps determine appropriate treatment approaches. **Acute wounds** result from surgery, trauma, or medical procedures and typically heal in predictable time frames. **Chronic**

wounds fail to heal within expected time periods, often due to underlying conditions that impair healing.

Wound depth classification describes tissue involvement:

- **Superficial** wounds affect only the epidermis
- **Partial-thickness** wounds extend into the dermis
- **Full-thickness** wounds extend through all skin layers into subcutaneous tissue
- **Deep** wounds may involve muscle, bone, or other structures

Wound assessment requires systematic evaluation of multiple characteristics. Measure length, width, and depth using appropriate tools. Note the wound bed appearance—healthy granulation tissue appears red and slightly bumpy, while necrotic tissue may be yellow, brown, or black.

Assess wound edges for signs of healing or complications. Healthy wound edges are pink and show signs of epithelialization (new skin growth). Undermining or tunneling indicates tissue destruction beyond the visible wound surface.

Drainage assessment includes amount, color, consistency, and odor. **Serous** drainage is clear and watery, **sanguineous** drainage contains blood, and **purulent** drainage indicates infection. Document drainage amount as scant, minimal, moderate, or copious based on dressing saturation.

Wound cleaning principles support healing while removing debris and bacteria. Clean from clean areas toward dirty areas to avoid spreading contamination. Use gentle pressure to avoid damaging fragile healing tissue. Normal saline is the preferred cleaning solution for most wounds.

Irrigation technique removes loose debris and bacteria more effectively than wiping. Use a 30-60 mL syringe with an 18-gauge needle or angiocatheter to generate appropriate pressure. Direct the stream at an angle to avoid forcing debris deeper into the wound.

Dressing Selection and Application

Choosing appropriate wound dressings requires understanding how different materials interact with wounds and support healing. The ideal dressing maintains a moist wound environment, absorbs excess drainage, protects from contamination, and allows for comfortable wear.

Moist wound healing principles guide modern wound care approaches. Wounds heal faster in moist environments compared to dry conditions. Moisture facilitates cell migration, enzyme activity, and tissue growth while reducing pain and scarring.

Gauze dressings remain useful for many wound types despite being considered traditional. Woven gauze provides absorption and can be impregnated with medications or solutions. Non-adherent gauze reduces tissue trauma during dressing changes. Use gauze dressings for wounds requiring frequent monitoring or those with heavy drainage.

Transparent film dressings provide moisture retention while allowing wound visualization. These thin, adhesive films work well for superficial wounds, IV sites, and protective barriers over intact skin. They're not appropriate for infected wounds or those with moderate to heavy drainage.

Hydrocolloid dressings contain gel-forming agents that create a moist environment while absorbing drainage. These opaque dressings can remain in place for several days and work well for pressure injuries and minor wounds. Remove carefully to avoid damaging fragile skin around wound edges.

Foam dressings provide excellent absorption while maintaining moisture balance. These dressings work well for wounds with moderate drainage and can be used under compression therapy. Many foam dressings have adhesive borders for secure attachment.

Hydrogel dressings provide moisture to dry wounds and can help soften necrotic tissue. These cooling, soothing dressings work well for painful wounds and burns. They require secondary dressings for attachment and protection.

Application techniques vary by dressing type but follow general principles. Clean hands thoroughly and use appropriate personal protective equipment. Clean the wound as needed before applying new dressings. Ensure dressings extend beyond wound edges to provide adequate protection.

Secure dressings appropriately without creating excessive tension that could impair circulation. Change dressings based on manufacturer recommendations, wound drainage, and patient comfort. Some dressings can remain in place for several days, while others require daily changes.

Drain Management

Surgical drains remove excess fluid and air from body cavities and wound sites, preventing complications and promoting healing. Understanding different drain types and proper management techniques ensures patient safety and optimal outcomes.

Drain purposes include removing blood, serum, and other fluids that could interfere with healing or create infection risks. Drains also help collapsed tissues re-expand and provide early warning of complications like bleeding or anastomotic leaks.

Passive drains rely on gravity and natural body movements to remove fluids. Penrose drains are soft rubber tubes that allow fluid to drain along their surface. These drains typically have safety pins to prevent migration and require frequent dressing changes to manage drainage.

Active drains use suction to remove fluids more effectively. Jackson-Pratt (JP) drains use squeezable bulb reservoirs to create negative pressure. Hemovac drains use spring-loaded chambers for continuous

200

suction. These closed systems reduce infection risk and allow accurate measurement of drainage.

Drain care principles focus on maintaining function while preventing complications. Keep drainage systems below the insertion site to promote gravity drainage. Maintain negative pressure in active drainage systems by compressing reservoirs after emptying.

Emptying procedures require sterile technique to prevent contamination. Empty drains when they're two-thirds full or according to facility schedules. Measure and record drainage amounts, noting color, consistency, and any unusual characteristics.

Clean the drainage spout with alcohol before and after emptying. Compress the reservoir completely before replacing the cap to reestablish negative pressure. Document drainage amount and characteristics according to facility protocols.

Monitoring for complications includes watching for signs of infection, drain displacement, or malfunction. Sudden increases or decreases in drainage may indicate complications. Purulent drainage, fever, or increased pain around the drain site may suggest infection.

Recognizing Infection vs. Normal Healing

Distinguishing between normal healing responses and wound infections requires understanding expected healing processes and concerning signs that require immediate attention. Early recognition and treatment of infections can prevent serious complications.

Normal healing signs include mild erythema around wound edges, minimal clear to slightly bloody drainage, and gradual wound closure. Some tenderness is normal, especially in the first few days after injury. Granulation tissue should appear red and bumpy as new blood vessels form.

Infection indicators include increasing erythema that extends beyond wound edges, purulent drainage with foul odor, increased pain or tenderness, and wound edge separation. Fever, elevated white blood cell count, and red streaking from the wound may indicate systemic infection requiring immediate medical attention.

Wound culture techniques help identify specific bacteria causing infections. Clean the wound with normal saline before obtaining culture specimens. Use sterile swabs to collect samples from deep within the wound, avoiding surface drainage or necrotic tissue that may not represent the true infection.

Antibiotic therapy requires appropriate selection based on culture results when possible. Topical antibiotics may be sufficient for superficial infections, while deeper or systemic infections require oral or intravenous antibiotics. Monitor patients for therapeutic response and adverse effects.

Infection prevention strategies include maintaining sterile technique during wound care, changing dressings appropriately, and ensuring adequate nutrition and hydration. Hand hygiene remains the most important factor in preventing healthcare-associated infections.

Case Study: Mrs. Johnson's Post-Operative Wound Complications

Mrs. Johnson, a 68-year-old woman with diabetes, underwent abdominal surgery for gallbladder removal five days ago. Her initial recovery was unremarkable, but now she's developing concerning changes in her surgical incision that require immediate nursing assessment and intervention.

Current presentation: Mrs. Johnson reports increased pain around her incision site, rating it 7/10 compared to 3/10 yesterday. The incision, which was previously well-approximated with minimal drainage, now shows 2 cm of separation at the center with moderate amounts of yellow-green drainage.

Assessment findings: The incision measures 15 cm in length with a 2 cm area of dehiscence (separation) in the center. Surrounding skin shows erythema extending 3 cm from the wound edges. The drainage has a foul odor and appears purulent. Mrs. Johnson's temperature is 101.8°F, her white blood cell count is elevated at 14,000, and her blood glucose is 285 mg/dL.

Risk factors contributing to complications:

- Diabetes affecting immune function and healing
- Elevated blood glucose providing favorable environment for bacterial growth
- Obesity increasing tension on the incision line
- Possible surgical site contamination during the procedure

Nursing interventions:

1. **Notify the surgeon immediately** about the wound dehiscence and signs of infection
2. **Obtain wound culture** using sterile technique before cleaning the wound
3. **Document wound characteristics** including measurements, drainage description, and surrounding skin condition
4. **Implement wound isolation precautions** to prevent spread of infection
5. **Monitor vital signs closely** for signs of systemic infection
6. **Coordinate blood glucose management** with endocrinology team to optimize healing

Treatment modifications: The surgeon ordered wound irrigation and debridement with packing to allow healing from the inside out. Antibiotic therapy was started based on culture results. Mrs. Johnson's diabetes management was intensified to maintain blood glucose below 180 mg/dL to support healing.

Case Study: Mr. Rodriguez's Pressure Injury Development

Mr. Rodriguez, a 78-year-old man admitted with pneumonia, has been bed-bound for several days due to weakness and breathing difficulties. Despite prevention efforts, he develops a Stage 2 pressure injury on his sacrum that requires immediate intervention to prevent progression.

Pressure injury characteristics: The sacral area shows a 3 cm x 2 cm area of partial-thickness skin loss with a shallow crater. The wound bed appears pink with minimal serous drainage. Surrounding skin shows some erythema but no induration or warmth.

Contributing factors:

- Prolonged bed rest due to respiratory illness
- Poor nutrition with albumin level of 2.8 g/dL
- Incontinence episodes creating moisture exposure
- Decreased mobility due to weakness and oxygen requirements

Prevention strategies implemented:

1. **Increase repositioning frequency** to every 1-2 hours with proper positioning techniques
2. **Upgrade to pressure-redistributing mattress** with alternating pressure capabilities
3. **Implement aggressive nutrition support** including protein supplements and dietitian consultation
4. **Manage incontinence proactively** with scheduled toileting and appropriate skin barriers
5. **Optimize pain management** to encourage mobility and position changes

Wound treatment plan: The pressure injury was treated with hydrocolloid dressing to maintain moist healing environment while protecting from further pressure and friction. The dressing was changed every 3-4 days unless drainage required more frequent changes.

Monitoring and outcomes: With aggressive prevention measures and appropriate wound care, Mr. Rodriguez's pressure injury showed signs of healing within one week. New epithelial tissue formed at the wound edges, and the wound bed remained pink and healthy throughout the healing process.

Case Study: Sarah's Diabetic Foot Ulcer Management

Sarah, a 52-year-old woman with poorly controlled diabetes, presents to the clinic with a foot ulcer that started as a small blister two weeks ago. The wound has progressively worsened despite her attempts at home care, highlighting the complexity of diabetic wound management.

Wound characteristics: The ulcer on the plantar surface of her right foot measures 2.5 cm x 1.8 cm x 0.8 cm deep. The wound bed contains both red granulation tissue and yellow fibrous tissue. Drainage is minimal but has a slight odor. Surrounding skin appears callused with some erythema.

Diabetic complications affecting healing:

- Poor glucose control with HbA1c of 10.2%
- Peripheral neuropathy reducing protective sensation
- Peripheral artery disease compromising circulation
- History of delayed healing with previous wounds

Comprehensive assessment:

1. **Vascular evaluation** including pulse assessment and ankle-brachial index
2. **Neurological testing** for protective sensation using monofilaments
3. **Infection assessment** including wound culture and blood work
4. **Glycemic control evaluation** with recent glucose logs and HbA1c
5. **Footwear assessment** to identify pressure points and friction areas

Treatment approach:

1. **Debridement** of necrotic tissue to promote healthy granulation
2. **Moisture-balancing dressing** changed every 2-3 days

3. **Offloading** with specialized footwear to reduce pressure on the ulcer
4. **Glucose optimization** through medication adjustments and dietary counseling
5. **Infection management** with topical antimicrobials based on culture results

Patient education priorities:

- Daily foot inspection techniques and what to report
- Proper wound care and dressing change procedures
- Importance of glucose control for healing
- Appropriate footwear selection and fit
- When to seek immediate medical attention

Long-term outcomes: With consistent treatment and improved glucose control, Sarah's ulcer showed progressive healing over 8 weeks. The key to success was addressing all factors affecting healing while providing comprehensive patient education to prevent recurrence.

Building Wound Care Expertise

Developing competence in skin and wound care requires understanding both the science of healing and the art of patient care. Each wound tells a story about the patient's overall health, healing capacity, and care needs. Your ability to read these stories and respond appropriately can significantly impact patient outcomes.

Evidence-based practice guides modern wound care decisions. Stay current with research on new dressing materials, treatment techniques, and prevention strategies. Many traditional practices (like using hydrogen peroxide or letting wounds "air dry") have been replaced by approaches that better support healing.

Interdisciplinary collaboration optimizes wound care outcomes. Work closely with wound care specialists, physicians, dietitians, and physical therapists to address all factors affecting healing. Each discipline brings unique expertise to complex wound management situations.

Documentation standards for wound care must be detailed and objective. Include wound measurements, descriptions of wound bed and edges, drainage characteristics, surrounding skin condition, and patient responses to treatment. Photographs can supplement written descriptions when permitted by facility policies.

Patient and family education promotes healing and prevents recurrence. Teach proper wound care techniques, signs of infection to report, and lifestyle modifications that support healing. Ensure patients understand the importance of following treatment recommendations and keeping follow-up appointments.

Protecting the Body's Fortress

Skin integrity and wound care represent fundamental aspects of nursing that affect every patient you'll care for. Your understanding of normal skin function, healing processes, and evidence-based interventions can prevent complications and promote optimal outcomes.

The complexity of wound healing requires nurses who understand not just the mechanics of dressing changes, but the physiological processes involved in repair and the multiple factors that can impair or enhance healing. Your role in protecting skin integrity and supporting wound healing makes you an essential advocate for patient safety and comfort.

Excellence in skin and wound care builds confidence and expertise that serves patients throughout their healing journeys. The prevention strategies you implement, the assessment skills you develop, and the treatment techniques you master contribute directly to patient outcomes and quality of life.

Key Learning Points

- **Understand skin structure and function** to recognize normal characteristics and identify problems early
- **Implement evidence-based pressure injury prevention** strategies for all at-risk patients
- **Master basic wound assessment** including measurement, description, and documentation techniques
- **Select appropriate dressings** based on wound characteristics and healing requirements
- **Recognize signs of infection** and differentiate them from normal healing responses
- **Provide proper drain management** including emptying, measuring, and monitoring for complications
- **Educate patients and families** about wound care techniques and prevention strategies
- **Collaborate with interdisciplinary teams** to address all factors affecting skin integrity and healing

Chapter 12: Pain Management and Comfort Measures

Pain touches every human life, yet it remains one of medicine's most complex and challenging aspects. The businessman who rates his post-surgical pain as 2/10 while tears stream down his face. The elderly woman who insists she's "fine" despite obvious discomfort with every movement. The teenager who dramatically claims 10/10 pain from what appears to be a minor injury. Each represents the deeply personal, subjective nature of pain that requires your skilled assessment and compassionate response.

Your role in pain management extends far beyond administering medications. You become a detective, uncovering the complex factors that contribute to each person's pain experience. You become an advocate, ensuring that pain relief remains a priority even in busy healthcare environments. You become a healer, using both pharmacological and non-pharmacological approaches to restore comfort and promote recovery.

Pain affects every aspect of healing—sleep, appetite, mobility, mood, and motivation to participate in care. Uncontrolled pain slows recovery, increases complications, and can lead to chronic pain conditions that persist long after initial injuries heal. Your understanding of pain principles and management strategies directly impacts patient outcomes and quality of life.

Understanding Pain

Pain serves as the body's warning system, alerting us to actual or potential tissue damage. However, this protective mechanism can become a problem when pain persists beyond its useful purpose or when conditions cause pain without clear tissue damage.

Pain's impact on healing affects multiple body systems and recovery processes. Uncontrolled pain increases stress hormone production, which can impair immune function and delay wound healing. Pain reduces deep breathing and mobility, increasing risks of pneumonia and blood clots. It interferes with sleep, which is essential for tissue repair and immune function (34).

Pain affects appetite and nutrition by reducing interest in food and interfering with normal digestive processes. Patients in pain often eat less, compromising their nutritional status just when their bodies need additional resources for healing. This creates a cycle where poor nutrition further impairs healing and pain control.

Mobility limitations from pain can lead to muscle weakness, joint stiffness, and cardiovascular deconditioning. Patients who avoid movement because of pain may develop complications that are more serious than their original conditions. Encouraging appropriate activity while managing pain becomes a delicate balancing act.

Mood and motivation suffer when pain is poorly controlled. Chronic pain is strongly associated with depression and anxiety, which can further reduce pain tolerance and complicate treatment. Patients may lose motivation to participate in therapies or self-care activities, slowing recovery and reducing independence.

Pain assessment frequency should occur regularly throughout your care. The American Pain Society recommends assessing pain as the "fifth sign" along with temperature, pulse, respiration, and blood pressure. For hospitalized patients experiencing pain, assessments should occur at least every 4 hours and before and after pain interventions.

Individual variations in pain experience require personalized approaches to assessment and management. Factors influencing pain include age, gender, cultural background, previous pain experiences, anxiety level, and personal coping strategies. What constitutes severe pain for one person may be manageable for another.

Pharmacologic Interventions

Understanding basic categories of pain medications helps you administer them safely and monitor for both therapeutic effects and adverse reactions. While you don't need to memorize every detail about specific drugs, you need enough knowledge to provide safe care and patient education.

Non-opioid analgesics form the foundation of many pain management plans. **Acetaminophen** provides pain relief and fever reduction without anti-inflammatory effects. It's generally well-tolerated but can cause liver damage with overdose or in patients with liver disease. Maximum daily dose for healthy adults is 4000 mg, but many facilities use 3000 mg as a safer limit.

Nonsteroidal anti-inflammatory drugs (NSAIDs) like ibuprofen, naproxen, and aspirin reduce pain and inflammation. These medications work by blocking enzymes that produce inflammatory substances. Common side effects include stomach upset, bleeding risk, and kidney problems, especially in elderly patients or those with kidney disease.

Opioid analgesics provide powerful pain relief for moderate to severe pain. Examples include morphine, oxycodone, hydrocodone, and fentanyl. These medications work by binding to opioid receptors in the brain and spinal cord, reducing pain perception and emotional response to pain.

Nursing considerations for opioids include monitoring respiratory status, as respiratory depression is the most serious potential side effect. Check respiratory rate and depth before administering opioids, especially for patients who are opioid-naive or receiving high doses. Oxygen saturation monitoring may also be appropriate.

Sedation assessment helps identify patients at risk for respiratory depression before it becomes life-threatening. Use a standardized sedation scale to evaluate consciousness level. Increasing sedation often precedes respiratory depression, making it an important early warning sign.

Common opioid side effects include constipation, nausea, drowsiness, and itching. Constipation occurs in most patients taking opioids regularly and should be prevented with bowel regimens including stool softeners, laxatives, and adequate fluid intake. Nausea often improves after a few days but may require antiemetic medications initially.

Addiction concerns affect many patients and healthcare providers but shouldn't prevent appropriate pain treatment. True addiction involves compulsive drug use despite harmful consequences and is relatively rare in patients receiving opioids for legitimate pain. Physical dependence and tolerance are normal physiological responses that differ from addiction.

Non-Pharmacologic Comfort Measures

Non-drug approaches to pain relief can be surprisingly effective and often work synergistically with medications to provide better comfort than either approach alone. These interventions have few side effects and can be used repeatedly without safety concerns.

Positioning modifications can significantly reduce pain from pressure, muscle tension, or joint stiffness. Support painful areas with pillows or cushions. Elevate swollen extremities to reduce pain from fluid accumulation. Change positions regularly to prevent new pressure points and muscle fatigue.

Heat therapy increases blood flow, relaxes muscles, and can provide significant pain relief for many conditions. Apply heat using heating pads, warm compresses, or warm baths for 15-20 minutes at a time. Always check skin temperature tolerance and inspect skin regularly to prevent burns, especially in patients with decreased sensation.

Cold therapy reduces inflammation, numbs painful areas, and can be particularly effective for acute injuries or inflammation. Apply cold using ice packs, cold compresses, or cool baths for 10-15 minutes at a time. Always protect skin with a barrier (towel or cloth) to prevent cold injury.

Massage therapy promotes relaxation, increases circulation, and may trigger release of natural pain-relieving substances. Simple hand, foot, or back massage can be performed by nurses or family members. Use gentle pressure and avoid areas with blood clots, infections, or recent surgery.

Relaxation techniques help patients manage pain by reducing muscle tension and anxiety. **Deep breathing exercises** involve slow, controlled breathing that activates the body's relaxation response. Guide patients to breathe in slowly through the nose, hold briefly, then exhale slowly through the mouth.

Progressive muscle relaxation involves systematically tensing and relaxing muscle groups throughout the body. Start with feet and work upward, holding tension for 5 seconds then releasing and noticing the contrast between tension and relaxation.

Guided imagery uses mental visualization to promote relaxation and pain relief. Help patients imagine peaceful, comfortable places or visualize healing occurring in their bodies. Recorded imagery sessions can be helpful for patients who have difficulty with self-directed visualization.

Distraction techniques redirect attention away from pain by engaging the mind in other activities. Music, television, reading, video games, or conversation can all provide distraction. The effectiveness often depends on matching the distraction to the patient's interests and cognitive abilities.

Environmental modifications create conditions that support comfort and relaxation. Reduce noise levels, adjust lighting to patient preference, maintain comfortable room temperature, and eliminate unpleasant odors. Sometimes simple changes like closing a door or dimming lights can significantly improve comfort.

Individualizing Pain Control

Pain is fundamentally subjective—only the person experiencing it can truly describe its characteristics and intensity. This subjectivity requires individualized approaches that account for personal, cultural, and medical factors affecting each patient's pain experience.

Believing patient reports forms the foundation of effective pain management. The American Pain Society emphasizes that pain is "what the patient says it is, when the patient says it is." This principle guides pain assessment and treatment decisions, recognizing that healthcare providers cannot accurately judge another person's pain.

Cultural influences on pain expression vary significantly among different groups. Some cultures encourage stoic responses to pain, viewing pain expression as weakness or lack of courage. Others support more expressive responses and expect healthcare providers to prioritize pain relief. Understanding these differences helps you provide culturally sensitive care.

Family involvement in pain management varies based on cultural norms and individual preferences. Some patients want family members involved in all pain-related decisions, while others prefer to maintain privacy about their pain experience. Ask patients about their preferences for family involvement.

Language barriers can complicate pain assessment and management. Use professional interpreters when possible, and be aware that pain descriptors may not translate directly between languages. Visual analog scales, faces pain scales, or numeric scales may work better than verbal descriptions for some patients.

Previous pain experiences influence current pain perception and coping strategies. Patients who have experienced severe pain before may have developed effective coping strategies, or they may have heightened anxiety about pain recurrence. Understanding pain history helps you anticipate needs and build on successful strategies.

Advocacy responsibilities include ensuring that patient pain concerns are heard and addressed appropriately. Speak up when pain seems inadequately treated, when patients express dissatisfaction with pain control, or when organizational factors interfere with appropriate pain management.

Documentation requirements for pain management should include pain scores, interventions used, patient responses, and any barriers to effective treatment. This documentation helps other healthcare providers understand what has and hasn't worked for each patient.

Special Considerations for End-of-Life Pain

Pain control becomes a primary goal in hospice and palliative care settings, where comfort takes precedence over other treatment considerations. Understanding the principles and approaches used in end-of-life care helps you provide compassionate care for dying patients.

Comfort as the primary goal means that pain relief takes priority over concerns about addiction, tolerance, or side effects that might be relevant in other situations. The focus shifts from preserving life to maintaining quality of life and dignity during the dying process.

Higher medication doses may be necessary to achieve adequate comfort in end-of-life situations. Patients may require doses that would be inappropriate in other circumstances, but the goal of comfort justifies these approaches when used by experienced practitioners.

Routes of administration may need modification as patients become unable to swallow medications. Sublingual, rectal, or transdermal routes can provide effective pain relief when oral administration is no longer possible. Some medications can be given through feeding tubes if present.

Breakthrough pain management addresses sudden increases in pain intensity that occur despite regularly scheduled medications. These episodes require rapid-acting medications and may indicate need for adjustments in baseline pain management regimens.

Family education and support help families understand pain management approaches and participate appropriately in comfort care. Families may need reassurance that appropriate pain medications don't hasten death and that keeping patients comfortable is a humane and necessary goal.

Case Study: Mr. Williams' Post-Surgical Pain Management

Mr. Williams, a 58-year-old construction worker, underwent major back surgery yesterday to repair herniated discs that had been causing severe chronic pain for months. He's now experiencing significant acute post-operative pain that requires careful assessment and management.

Current pain status: Mr. Williams rates his pain as 8/10, describing it as "sharp and burning" in his lower back with radiation down his right leg. He says the pain is worse than before surgery and worries that the operation didn't help. He appears restless and has difficulty finding comfortable positions.

Pain management orders:

- Morphine PCA (patient-controlled analgesia) 1 mg every 6 minutes, maximum 10 mg per hour
- Ibuprofen 600 mg every 6 hours around the clock
- Ice packs to surgical site for 20 minutes every 2 hours
- Position changes every 2 hours with assistance

Assessment findings: Mr. Williams has used 8 mg of morphine in the past hour but reports minimal relief. His vital signs show mild elevations in blood pressure (148/92) and heart rate (98) consistent with pain response. He's alert and oriented with respiratory rate of 16 and oxygen saturation of 96%.

Nursing interventions:

216

1. **Reassess pain thoroughly** using PQRST method to understand pain characteristics and compare to pre-operative pain
2. **Review PCA effectiveness** by checking usage patterns and patient understanding of device operation
3. **Ensure around-the-clock medications** are being given as scheduled, not just when requested
4. **Implement non-pharmacological measures** including positioning, ice application, and relaxation techniques
5. **Educate about expected recovery** and normal post-operative pain patterns versus concerning symptoms

Collaborative care: The nurse contacted the surgeon to report inadequate pain control despite maximum PCA usage. The physician increased the PCA dose to 1.5 mg and added acetaminophen 1000 mg every 6 hours. Physical therapy was consulted for positioning and mobility guidance.

Follow-up outcomes: With medication adjustments and consistent use of non-pharmacological measures, Mr. Williams' pain decreased to 4-5/10 within 24 hours. He began participating in physical therapy and reported improved confidence about his recovery prospects.

Case Study: Mrs. Chen's Chronic Pain Challenge

Mrs. Chen, a 72-year-old retired seamstress, has been living with chronic arthritis pain for over 10 years. She's now hospitalized for pneumonia, but her chronic pain is significantly complicating her recovery and affecting her mood and participation in care.

Chronic pain history: Mrs. Chen takes a daily long-acting opioid (oxycodone extended-release 20 mg twice daily) plus immediate-release oxycodone 5 mg every 4 hours as needed for breakthrough pain. At home, she manages reasonably well with this regimen plus heat therapy and gentle exercises.

Current complications: The stress of illness has increased Mrs. Chen's pain levels, and the hospital environment makes it difficult to use her usual coping strategies. She's reluctant to ask for pain medication, saying she doesn't want to "bother" the nurses. Her pain is now 7/10 most of the time, and she's becoming increasingly withdrawn.

Cultural considerations: Mrs. Chen comes from a culture that emphasizes stoicism and avoiding complaints. She believes that pain is part of aging and that she should "bear it quietly." Her family supports this view and seems uncomfortable when she expresses pain.

Nursing approaches:

1. **Establish trust** by spending time with Mrs. Chen and acknowledging her pain as real and important
2. **Educate about pain treatment** and explain that managing pain will help her recover from pneumonia faster
3. **Maintain home medication regimen** as much as possible while adding treatments for increased pain
4. **Adapt comfort measures** to hospital environment using heating pads, positioning aids, and quiet periods
5. **Involve family appropriately** in supporting pain management while respecting cultural values

Outcomes: With consistent pain management and cultural sensitivity, Mrs. Chen's pain decreased to manageable levels. She became more willing to participate in respiratory therapy and ambulation, leading to faster recovery from pneumonia and earlier discharge home.

Case Study: Jamie's Adolescent Pain Experience

Jamie, a 16-year-old high school athlete, sustained a serious ankle fracture during soccer practice and underwent surgical repair. Pain management for adolescents requires special considerations regarding development, communication, and family involvement.

Unique challenges: Jamie is devastated about missing the remainder of soccer season and worried about college scholarship opportunities. The physical pain is compounded by emotional distress about the injury's impact on future plans. Jamie alternates between acting "tough" and becoming tearful about the situation.

Family dynamics: Jamie's parents are concerned about opioid addiction risk and prefer to limit pain medication use. They express beliefs that Jamie should "tough it out" and that pain medication might interfere with healing. However, they're also distressed seeing Jamie in obvious discomfort.

Developmental considerations: As an adolescent, Jamie wants to maintain some independence and control over treatment decisions while still needing parental support. Body image concerns about scarring and future athletic ability add to the emotional burden of injury.

Nursing strategies:

1. **Involve Jamie in decision-making** while respecting parental concerns and legal requirements
2. **Provide age-appropriate education** about pain management, addiction risks, and healing processes
3. **Address emotional aspects** of injury including grief over lost opportunities and fears about recovery
4. **Encourage appropriate coping strategies** including connection with teammates and focus on rehabilitation goals
5. **Balance independence and support** by allowing Jamie choices while ensuring adequate supervision

Family education priorities:

- Difference between appropriate pain treatment and addiction risk
- Importance of adequate pain control for healing and rehabilitation
- Signs of concerning behaviors versus normal adolescent responses to major injury
- Ways to support Jamie's emotional adjustment to injury

Long-term planning: With appropriate pain management and emotional support, Jamie successfully completed rehabilitation and returned to soccer the following season. The family gained understanding about appropriate pain treatment and became advocates for balanced approaches to adolescent pain management.

Building Pain Management Expertise

Developing competence in pain management requires understanding both the science of pain and the art of comfort care. Each patient brings unique experiences, expectations, and needs that require individualized approaches to assessment and treatment.

Evidence-based practice guides modern pain management approaches. Stay current with research on new medications, non-pharmacological interventions, and assessment tools. Many traditional beliefs about pain (such as addiction fears or tolerance concerns) have been challenged by newer evidence.

Interdisciplinary collaboration optimizes pain management outcomes. Work closely with physicians, pharmacists, physical therapists, and pain specialists to address all aspects of pain experience. Each discipline brings unique perspectives and interventions to complex pain situations.

Patient and family education promotes understanding and cooperation with pain management plans. Teach about pain assessment tools, medication expectations, non-pharmacological techniques, and when to report concerns. Address fears and misconceptions that may interfere with effective treatment.

Self-care considerations help you maintain empathy and effectiveness when caring for patients in pain. Watching people suffer can be emotionally draining, and the pressure to "fix" pain can create frustration when relief is difficult to achieve. Develop healthy coping strategies and seek support when needed.

Restoring Comfort, Promoting Healing

Pain management represents one of nursing's most fundamental responsibilities and greatest challenges. Your ability to assess pain accurately, implement appropriate interventions, and advocate for adequate treatment directly impacts patient outcomes and satisfaction with care.

The complexity of pain requires nurses who understand not just the mechanics of medication administration, but the physiological, psychological, and social factors that influence pain experience. Your role in promoting comfort extends beyond technical skills to include compassion, advocacy, and individualized care that respects each person's unique pain experience.

Excellence in pain management builds trust and therapeutic relationships that benefit all aspects of patient care. When patients feel confident that their pain concerns are heard and addressed, they're more likely to participate actively in their recovery and report other important symptoms or concerns.

Key Learning Points

- **Understand pain's impact** on healing, mood, mobility, and overall recovery to prioritize appropriate management
- **Master pain assessment techniques** including use of appropriate scales and systematic evaluation methods
- **Implement safe medication practices** for both opioid and non-opioid analgesics with attention to side effects and monitoring
- **Use non-pharmacological interventions** effectively as adjuncts to medication therapy for enhanced comfort
- **Individualize pain management approaches** based on cultural, developmental, and personal factors
- **Advocate for adequate pain treatment** while addressing patient and family concerns about medication use
- **Document pain management comprehensively** including assessment findings, interventions, and patient responses
- **Collaborate with interdisciplinary teams** to optimize comfort and promote recovery for all patients

Chapter 13: Oxygenation – Basics of Respiratory Care

The human body depends on oxygen like a car depends on gasoline. Without it, everything stops working. Yet many new nurses feel uncertain about respiratory care, wondering if they're doing enough or recognizing problems early. This chapter will change that uncertainty into confidence.

Understanding Oxygenation Assessment

Your assessment skills determine how quickly you spot respiratory problems. A patient's breathing tells a story—you just need to know how to read it.

Normal respiratory patterns show us what healthy looks like: 12-20 breaths per minute in adults, quiet and effortless breathing, and oxygen saturation levels between 95-100%. The patient talks in full sentences without gasping, and their color remains pink and healthy (1).

Impaired oxygenation presents differently. Watch for respiratory rates outside the normal range, shortness of breath during minimal activity, and the use of accessory muscles—those neck and shoulder muscles that shouldn't be working hard during quiet breathing. Cyanosis, that bluish tint around the lips and fingernails, signals severe oxygen deprivation (2).

Case Example 1: Maria, a 68-year-old post-operative patient, seemed fine during morning rounds. By afternoon, she was breathing 28 times per minute, using her neck muscles to breathe, and complained of feeling "winded" just talking. Her oxygen saturation had dropped to 89%. These signs pointed to developing respiratory distress that required immediate intervention.

Lung sounds provide another assessment tool. **Clear lung sounds** indicate good air movement. **Crackles** sound like cellophane crinkling and often suggest fluid in the lungs. **Wheezes** create a high-pitched whistling sound, typically indicating narrowed airways from conditions like asthma or bronchospasm (3).

Case Example 2: John, a 55-year-old with heart failure, developed fine crackles in his lower lung fields. His oxygen saturation remained normal at 96%, but the crackles indicated early fluid accumulation. Early recognition allowed for medication adjustments before his condition worsened.

Oxygen Delivery Systems

Different patients need different amounts of oxygen support. Understanding these devices helps you match the right tool to each patient's needs.

Nasal cannula delivers 1-6 liters per minute of oxygen, providing 24-44% oxygen concentration. It's comfortable for long-term use and allows patients to eat and talk normally. Check that the prongs sit properly in the nostrils and that the tubing isn't kinked (4).

Simple face masks deliver 5-10 liters per minute, providing 35-50% oxygen concentration. They work well for patients needing higher oxygen levels than a nasal cannula can provide. Ensure the mask fits snugly but comfortably over the nose and mouth (5).

Non-rebreather masks deliver the highest concentration of oxygen without mechanical ventilation—up to 95% oxygen concentration with flow rates of 10-15 liters per minute. The reservoir bag must stay inflated to work properly. These masks are for patients in significant respiratory distress (6).

Safety considerations matter enormously with oxygen therapy. Oxygen supports combustion, making fire hazards deadly serious. Post "No Smoking" signs, remove potential ignition sources, and educate patients and families about these risks. High-flow oxygen can dry nasal passages, so humidification prevents discomfort and bleeding (7).

Case Example 3: Sarah, a 45-year-old smoker admitted with pneumonia, initially received 2 liters of oxygen via nasal cannula. Her oxygen saturation remained at 88% despite the supplemental oxygen. Switching to a simple face mask at 6 liters per minute brought her saturation to 94%. The key was recognizing when one device wasn't providing adequate support and escalating appropriately.

Positioning and Breathing Techniques

Simple interventions often produce remarkable results. Proper positioning and breathing techniques can significantly improve a patient's respiratory status.

High Fowler's position (sitting upright at 60-90 degrees) allows gravity to help the diaphragm move more efficiently. This position works particularly well for patients with heart failure, pneumonia, or any condition causing shortness of breath (8).

Deep breathing exercises prevent complications like pneumonia and atelectasis. Teach patients to take slow, deep breaths, hold for a few seconds, then exhale completely. This technique helps expand lung tissue and clear secretions (9).

Incentive spirometry provides measurable goals for deep breathing. Show patients how to seal their lips around the mouthpiece, breathe in slowly and deeply to raise the ball or piston, hold for 3-5 seconds, then exhale. Encourage use every hour while awake (10).

Airway Management Fundamentals

Keeping airways clear prevents respiratory complications. Your role includes helping patients mobilize secretions and recognizing when they need additional support.

Encouraging effective coughing helps patients clear secretions naturally. Teach the "huff" technique: take a deep breath, hold briefly, then force air out quickly while saying "huff." This technique moves secretions without the strain of traditional coughing (11).

Hydration plays a crucial role in thinning secretions. Encourage fluid intake unless contraindicated. Thinner secretions move more easily, preventing plugging of airways (12).

Recognizing when to escalate protects patients from deterioration. Call for help when patients show signs of severe distress: oxygen saturation below 90% despite supplemental oxygen, extreme difficulty breathing, confusion or altered mental status, or inability to speak in full sentences (13).

Signs That Demand Immediate Action

Some respiratory changes signal medical emergencies. Recognizing these signs and responding quickly can save lives.

Severe hypoxemia (oxygen saturation below 85%) requires immediate intervention. Don't wait—increase oxygen delivery and call for help immediately (14).

Acute respiratory distress shows itself through accessory muscle use, inability to speak in full sentences, and extreme anxiety. These patients need rapid assessment and likely intubation (15).

Changes in mental status from hypoxia include confusion, agitation, or decreased responsiveness. The brain suffers when oxygen levels drop, making these changes ominous signs (16).

Your response protocol should include: staying calm, increasing oxygen delivery as ordered, positioning the patient upright, calling for immediate help (rapid response team or physician), and preparing for possible intubation or other emergency interventions.

Practical Application Scenarios

Let's test your understanding with realistic situations you'll encounter.

Scenario 1: A patient with mild shortness of breath has an oxygen saturation of 91%. They're currently on room air. What oxygen delivery device would you choose?

Answer: Start with a nasal cannula at 2 liters per minute. This provides gentle oxygen support while allowing comfort and mobility.

Scenario 2: Teaching a post-operative patient to use an incentive spirometer. What steps would you include?

Answer: Explain the purpose, demonstrate proper technique, have them practice with coaching, set realistic goals (starting with their current best effort), and encourage hourly use while awake.

Scenario 3: A patient's oxygen saturation drops to 88% despite 4 liters via nasal cannula. What's your next step?

Answer: Switch to a simple face mask at 6-8 liters per minute, position them upright, assess for other causes of hypoxemia, and notify the physician of the change.

Building Your Assessment Skills

Respiratory assessment becomes intuitive with practice. Start with the basics: observe breathing patterns, check oxygen saturation, listen to lung sounds, and assess the patient's ability to speak comfortably.

Document your findings clearly. Instead of writing "patient appears short of breath," write "patient breathing 24 times per minute, using accessory muscles, oxygen saturation 90% on 2L nasal cannula, speaks in 3-4 word sentences."

Trust your instincts. If something seems wrong, it probably is. New nurses often worry about "bothering" doctors, but patient safety always comes first. A skilled nurse's observations provide crucial information for medical decision-making.

Bridging to Advanced Care

Understanding basic respiratory care prepares you for more complex interventions. You'll build on these foundations as you learn about mechanical ventilation, arterial blood gas interpretation, and advanced airway management.

These fundamental skills—assessment, oxygen delivery, positioning, and recognizing distress—form the cornerstone of respiratory nursing care. Master these basics, and you'll provide excellent care while building confidence for more advanced challenges.

Key Learning Points:

- Normal respiratory assessment parameters guide your baseline understanding
- Different oxygen delivery devices serve specific patient needs and clinical situations
- Proper positioning and breathing techniques provide simple but effective interventions
- Early recognition of respiratory distress prevents patient deterioration
- Clear documentation and communication ensure continuity of care

Chapter 14: Cultural and Psychosocial Considerations in Care

Healthcare happens between human beings, not just between a nurse and a medical condition. Every patient brings their culture, beliefs, fears, and life experiences into the hospital room. Understanding these factors transforms good technical care into healing relationships.

The Foundation of Holistic Care

Holistic nursing means seeing the whole person, not just the diagnosis. Physical symptoms often connect to emotional, cultural, or spiritual concerns. A patient's chest pain might stem from anxiety about family finances. Their reluctance to take medication might reflect cultural beliefs about Western medicine.

Physical care addresses symptoms, monitors vital signs, and manages treatments. **Emotional care** recognizes fear, grief, and uncertainty. **Cultural care** respects different ways of understanding health and illness. **Spiritual care** honors whatever gives patients meaning and hope (17).

This approach doesn't require you to be everything to everyone. Instead, it asks you to see each patient as a unique individual with their own needs, preferences, and ways of understanding their experience.

Cultural Competence in Action

Cultural competence isn't about memorizing facts about different ethnic groups. It's about approaching each patient with curiosity, respect, and openness to learning.

Ask, don't assume. Instead of guessing what a patient might prefer based on their appearance or name, ask directly. "Are there any cultural or religious practices that are important to you during your hospital stay?" opens the door for meaningful conversation (18).

Respect dietary needs. Food often carries deep cultural and religious significance. A Muslim patient might need to know if medications contain pork products. A Hindu patient might prefer vegetarian meals. These aren't just preferences—they're expressions of deeply held beliefs (19).

Understand family dynamics. In some cultures, family members make medical decisions collectively. In others, specific family members (like the eldest son) hold decision-making authority. Don't assume Western individualistic approaches apply to everyone (20).

Case Example 1: Mrs. Chen, a 72-year-old Chinese immigrant, seemed anxious and withdrawn during her cardiac catheterization preparation. When asked about her concerns, she revealed that her family hadn't been told about the procedure. In her culture, serious medical information is often shared with family members first, who then decide what to tell the patient. Working with the social worker and interpreter, the team included her family in the discussion, which significantly reduced her anxiety and improved her cooperation with care.

Language barriers require more than translation. Cultural concepts don't always translate directly. Work with professional interpreters, not family members, for medical discussions. Family interpreters might filter information to protect the patient or might not understand medical terminology (21).

Spiritual Care as Part of Healing

Spirituality encompasses formal religion, personal beliefs about meaning and purpose, and connections to something greater than oneself. For many patients, spiritual concerns become more urgent during illness.

Recognize spiritual needs. Listen for statements like "Why is this happening to me?" or "I don't know how to get through this." These often signal spiritual distress, not just emotional upset (22).

Facilitate spiritual support. You don't need to provide spiritual counseling yourself. Instead, connect patients with chaplains, their own religious leaders, or spiritual care resources. Ask, "Would you like me to contact a chaplain or your religious leader?" (23).

Respect religious practices. Some patients need to pray at specific times, face certain directions, or follow particular dietary laws. Others might want religious objects nearby or specific rituals performed. These practices often provide comfort and hope during frightening times (24).

Case Example 2: Ahmed, a 34-year-old Muslim man recovering from surgery, became increasingly agitated as evening approached. His nurse noticed he kept looking toward the window and checking the time. When asked about his concerns, he explained that he needed to pray but wasn't sure which direction faced Mecca. The nurse contacted the chaplain, who helped determine the correct direction and provided a prayer rug. Ahmed's anxiety decreased significantly, and he became more cooperative with his care plan.

Providing Psychosocial Support

Illness creates vulnerability. Patients lose control over their bodies, their schedules, and sometimes their futures. Your emotional support can significantly impact their healing process.

Active listening means giving your full attention. Put down your phone, make eye contact, and focus on what the patient is saying. Sometimes patients need to tell their story more than they need medical intervention (25).

Therapeutic presence involves being genuinely present with patients during difficult moments. You don't need to have all the answers. Sometimes sitting quietly while a patient cries or expressing concern for their worry provides more comfort than any medication (26).

Validate emotions. Statements like "It makes sense that you're scared" or "Many people feel overwhelmed in this situation" help patients feel understood rather than judged. Avoid minimizing their concerns with phrases like "Don't worry" or "Everything will be fine" (27).

Connect patients with resources. Social workers, support groups, chaplains, and mental health professionals extend your ability to provide comprehensive care. Don't hesitate to make these referrals— they're part of good nursing practice (28).

Mental Health in Hospital Settings

Medical illness often triggers anxiety and depression. Patients facing cancer diagnoses, chronic conditions, or significant lifestyle changes need mental health support alongside medical treatment.

Recognize symptoms. Anxiety might appear as restlessness, rapid breathing, or excessive worry about procedures. Depression might show as withdrawal, hopelessness, or loss of interest in activities. Both conditions can interfere with healing (29).

Respond appropriately. Acknowledge what you observe: "I notice you seem worried about tomorrow's procedure. Can you tell me what's concerning you?" This opens conversation without making assumptions (30).

Know when to refer. Patients expressing thoughts of self-harm, severe depression, or anxiety that interferes with medical care need professional mental health evaluation. Don't try to handle these situations alone (31).

Case Example 3: Jennifer, a 28-year-old new mother admitted with postpartum complications, burst into tears during routine medication administration. She expressed feeling overwhelmed, guilty about being away from her baby, and worried about being a "bad mother." The nurse spent time listening, validated her feelings as normal responses to a difficult situation, and arranged for social work consultation. The social worker connected Jennifer with postpartum support resources and counseling services, which helped her cope with both her medical condition and her emotional distress.

Communicating Across Differences

Effective communication bridges cultural, linguistic, and social differences. Your approach can either build trust or create barriers.

Use clear, simple language. Avoid medical jargon even with patients who speak English as a first language. Stress and illness make complex information harder to process (32).

Check for understanding. Ask patients to explain back what you've told them. This reveals misunderstandings before they become problems. "Can you tell me how you'll take this medication at home?" works better than "Do you understand?" (33).

Be patient with questions. Patients from different cultural backgrounds might need more time to process information or might have different ways of expressing concerns. Cultural norms about authority figures might make some patients reluctant to ask questions (34).

Respect different communication styles. Some cultures value direct communication, while others prefer indirect approaches. Some patients want detailed medical information, while others prefer broader explanations. Adjust your style to match their preferences (35).

Addressing Bias and Promoting Equity

Healthcare disparities reflect systemic problems, but individual nurses can make a difference through conscious attention to bias and advocacy for all patients.

Examine your assumptions. We all have unconscious biases based on race, age, gender, socioeconomic status, and other factors.

Regularly question whether these biases influence your care decisions (36).

Advocate for equitable care. Ensure all patients receive appropriate attention, pain management, and respect regardless of their background. Speak up when you notice disparities in treatment (37).

Support vulnerable populations. Patients with limited English proficiency, those without insurance, and those from marginalized communities often need extra advocacy. Your voice can help ensure they receive appropriate care (38).

Building Cultural Bridges

Healthcare works best when patients and providers understand each other. Your role includes building bridges across cultural differences.

Show genuine interest. Ask patients about their preferences, traditions, and concerns. Most people appreciate sincere interest in their background and experiences (39).

Learn from patients. Every patient teaches you something about their culture, their experiences, or their perspectives on health and illness. Approach each interaction as a learning opportunity (40).

Adapt your care. When possible, modify your approach to accommodate cultural preferences. This might mean adjusting visiting hours for large extended families, providing same-gender caregivers, or coordinating care around religious observances (41).

The Ripple Effect of Compassionate Care

Your cultural sensitivity and psychosocial support create ripples that extend far beyond the hospital stay. Patients who feel understood and respected often have better outcomes, higher satisfaction, and more trust in healthcare systems.

Family members observe how you treat their loved ones. Your compassionate care can change their entire family's relationship with healthcare. Other staff members learn from your example, creating a more inclusive environment for all patients.

Closing Reflection: Every patient who enters your care brings a lifetime of experiences, beliefs, and relationships. Your technical skills might heal their bodies, but your cultural sensitivity and emotional support heal their spirits. In a world that often feels divided, healthcare offers opportunities to build bridges of understanding and compassion. When you honor each patient's unique background and respond to their deepest fears with genuine care, you practice nursing at its highest level.

Key Learning Points:

- Holistic care addresses physical, emotional, cultural, and spiritual needs simultaneously
- Cultural competence requires curiosity, respect, and willingness to learn from patients
- Spiritual care connects patients with sources of meaning and hope during illness
- Mental health support often determines how well patients cope with medical conditions
- Effective communication bridges differences and builds therapeutic relationships

Chapter 15: Caring for Older Adults and Patients with Special Needs

The 85-year-old woman in room 312 isn't just an elderly patient with hip fracture—she's a retired teacher who raised five children, survived the loss of her husband, and maintains her own apartment. The 30-year-old man with developmental disabilities isn't defined by his diagnosis—he has preferences, relationships, and dignity that deserve respect. This chapter explores how to provide excellent care for patients whose needs require special consideration.

Understanding Geriatric Care Principles

Aging brings predictable changes that affect how you provide care. Understanding these changes helps you adapt your approach without making assumptions about individual capabilities.

Age-related changes occur gradually and vary significantly among individuals. Vision might become less sharp, hearing might diminish, and mobility might slow. Skin becomes thinner and more fragile. Memory might become less reliable, and processing new information might take longer (42).

Avoid ageism in your practice. Not all older adults are confused, weak, or incapable. Many maintain sharp minds, active lifestyles, and independence well into their 90s. Assess each patient individually rather than making assumptions based on age (43).

Adjust your communication for age-related changes. Speak clearly and face patients when talking to help with lip reading. Use good lighting and large print materials for visual impairments. Allow extra time for processing information and making decisions (44).

Case Example 1: Mr. Peterson, 78 years old, was admitted for cardiac monitoring after chest pain. The day nurse rushed through medication teaching, speaking quickly and facing away while preparing injections. Mr. Peterson appeared confused and asked the same questions repeatedly. The evening nurse noticed he wore hearing aids and wasn't wearing his glasses. She spoke slowly, faced him directly, made sure he wore his glasses, and provided written instructions in large print. Mr. Peterson's "confusion" disappeared, and he demonstrated perfect understanding of his medications and discharge instructions.

Fall Prevention and Safety

Falls represent the leading cause of injury among older adults. Your vigilance and interventions can prevent devastating consequences.

Assess fall risk systematically. Look for factors like muscle weakness, balance problems, medication side effects, cognitive impairment, previous falls, and environmental hazards. Use standardized fall risk assessment tools to guide your evaluation (45).

Implement prevention strategies based on individual risk factors. Keep call lights within reach, ensure adequate lighting, clear pathways of obstacles, and provide non-slip socks. Consider bed alarms or chair alarms for high-risk patients (46).

Medication management requires special attention. Older adults metabolize medications differently, making them more susceptible to side effects. Sedatives, blood pressure medications, and diuretics can increase fall risk. Monitor for dizziness, confusion, or unsteadiness (47).

Case Example 2: Mrs. Williams, 82 years old, was admitted for pneumonia treatment. Her fall risk assessment revealed previous falls, mild cognitive impairment, and medications that could cause dizziness. The nursing team implemented multiple interventions: bed alarm, hourly rounding, bathroom schedule to prevent rushing, and coordination with physical therapy for mobility assessment. Despite her high-risk factors, Mrs. Williams remained fall-free during her five-day stay.

Managing Polypharmacy Concerns

Older adults often take multiple medications, creating complex interactions and increased side effects. Your medication management skills can prevent serious complications.

Understand polypharmacy risks. Taking multiple medications increases the likelihood of drug interactions, adverse effects, and medication errors. Older adults metabolize drugs differently, making them more sensitive to medication effects (48).

Monitor for side effects that might not be obvious. Confusion might result from medication interactions rather than dementia. Falls might be caused by blood pressure medications rather than balance problems. Appetite changes might reflect medication side effects rather than depression (49).

Coordinate with pharmacy and physicians to review medication regimens regularly. Question medications that seem inappropriate for elderly patients or that duplicate effects of other medications (50).

Dementia and Delirium Care

Cognitive impairment affects how patients experience healthcare. Understanding the difference between chronic conditions like dementia and acute conditions like delirium guides your interventions.

Dementia develops gradually and represents permanent changes in memory, thinking, and behavior. Patients with dementia might not remember recent events but might recall distant memories clearly. They might become confused about where they are or who you are (51).

Delirium appears suddenly and represents acute confusion often caused by infection, medication changes, or other medical conditions. Unlike dementia, delirium can often be reversed by treating the underlying cause (52).

Communication strategies for cognitive impairment include using simple, clear language, maintaining eye contact, and speaking slowly.

Introduce yourself each time you enter the room. Use familiar objects or photographs to provide comfort and orientation (53).

Maintain routines when possible. Patients with dementia often function better with predictable schedules and familiar activities. Reduce environmental stimuli that might cause confusion or agitation (54).

Case Example 3: Mr. Martinez, 79 years old with mild dementia, became increasingly agitated during his second hospital day. He kept trying to leave his room, saying he needed to "get home to feed the cats." Instead of restraining him or arguing about reality, his nurse acknowledged his concern and redirected his attention to familiar activities. She provided a photo of his family, played his favorite music, and arranged for his daughter to visit during times when he became most restless. His agitation decreased significantly, and he required no sedative medications.

Caring for Patients with Sensory Impairments

Vision and hearing impairments affect how patients interact with their environment and healthcare providers. Simple accommodations can dramatically improve their experience.

Vision impairments range from mild decreases in acuity to complete blindness. Always announce yourself when entering the room. Describe what you're doing before you do it. Keep personal items in consistent locations so patients can find them (55).

Hearing impairments might be mild, severe, or complete. Face patients when speaking, use gestures and facial expressions, and write important information when necessary. Don't assume patients can read lips—this skill varies significantly among individuals (56).

Environmental modifications help patients navigate safely. Ensure adequate lighting, reduce background noise, and remove obstacles from pathways. Use contrasting colors to help patients distinguish between objects (57).

Developmental and Intellectual Disabilities

Patients with developmental disabilities bring unique strengths and challenges to healthcare settings. Your approach can either support their dignity and autonomy or create unnecessary barriers.

Person-first language respects individual dignity. Say "person with intellectual disability" rather than "mentally retarded person." Focus on the individual, not the disability (58).

Involve caregivers appropriately. Many adults with developmental disabilities have support persons who understand their needs, preferences, and communication styles. Include these individuals in care planning while respecting the patient's autonomy (59).

Adapt your communication to the patient's comprehension level. Use simple language, concrete examples, and visual aids when helpful. Allow extra time for processing information and making decisions (60).

Respect decision-making capacity. Many patients with developmental disabilities can make their own healthcare decisions. Don't assume lack of capacity based on diagnosis alone. Assess each patient's ability to understand information and express preferences (61).

Advocacy and Inclusion

Vulnerable populations often face discrimination or receive substandard care. Your advocacy can ensure all patients receive excellent treatment.

Speak up when you notice disparities in care. Patients with disabilities, older adults, or those with limited English proficiency might receive less attention or respect. Your voice can make a difference (62).

Challenge stereotypes among staff members. Educate colleagues about the capabilities and needs of patients with special requirements. Model respectful, inclusive care in your daily practice (63).

Connect patients with resources. Social workers, discharge planners, and community organizations can provide ongoing support. Don't assume patients have adequate resources or support systems (64).

Creating Inclusive Care Environments

The physical and social environment significantly impacts how patients with special needs experience healthcare.

Physical modifications might include better lighting, reduced noise, clear signage, and accessible equipment. Simple changes can make environments more welcoming and functional (65).

Staff education improves care quality. Training programs about cultural competence, disability awareness, and age-specific care help all staff members provide better service (66).

Family involvement often enhances care quality. Families understand patient preferences, routines, and needs better than healthcare providers. Include them in care planning and decision-making when appropriate (67).

Building Therapeutic Relationships

Patients with special needs often form strong attachments to healthcare providers who treat them with respect and understanding. These relationships can significantly impact health outcomes.

Consistency in caregivers helps build trust and understanding. When possible, assign the same nurses to patients with dementia, developmental disabilities, or complex social situations (68).

Patience allows patients to communicate their needs and preferences. Rushing through interactions often creates anxiety and misunderstanding. Allow extra time for patients who need it (69).

Dignity should guide every interaction. Patients with special needs often face discrimination or condescension. Your respectful approach can restore their confidence in healthcare systems (70).

Preparing for Discharge

Patients with special needs often require complex discharge planning. Your early involvement can prevent readmissions and ensure successful transitions.

Assess home environment and support systems. Patients with mobility limitations need accessible housing. Those with cognitive impairments need reliable caregivers. Identify potential problems early (71).

Coordinate services before discharge. Home healthcare, medical equipment, transportation, and follow-up appointments require advance planning. Social workers and discharge planners can help coordinate these services (72).

Educate caregivers about ongoing care needs. Family members and professional caregivers need clear instructions about medications, monitoring, and when to seek help (73).

The Broader Impact of Inclusive Care

Your approach to patients with special needs reflects your values and influences your colleagues. Inclusive care creates better outcomes for individuals and improves healthcare systems overall.

When you advocate for an elderly patient's dignity, you influence how your colleagues view aging. When you communicate effectively with a patient with developmental disabilities, you demonstrate that all patients deserve respect and quality care. When you adapt your approach for cultural differences, you create a more welcoming environment for diverse populations.

Reflective Insights: Healthcare at its best serves everyone with equal dedication and respect. Patients with special needs often test our patience, challenge our assumptions, and require extra effort. Yet these same patients often teach us the most about resilience, dignity, and the human spirit. Your willingness to adapt your care, advocate for inclusion, and see beyond diagnoses to the person underneath creates healing that extends far beyond medical treatment. In a profession dedicated to caring for the vulnerable, your special attention to those with the greatest needs represents nursing at its most noble.

Key Learning Points:

- Age-related changes require care adaptations but don't define individual capabilities
- Fall prevention strategies must address multiple risk factors simultaneously
- Cognitive impairment affects communication but doesn't eliminate patient dignity
- Sensory impairments require environmental modifications and communication adjustments
- Developmental disabilities call for person-centered approaches and appropriate support
- Advocacy ensures vulnerable populations receive equitable treatment and resources

Chapter 16: Care at the End of Life

Death remains the most difficult aspect of healthcare for many nurses. The monitors stop beeping, the breathing ceases, and families face their worst fears. Yet for nurses willing to embrace this sacred responsibility, end-of-life care offers opportunities for profound meaning and healing. This chapter explores how to provide compassionate support during life's final chapter.

Understanding End-of-Life Care

End-of-life care shifts focus from cure to comfort, from fighting disease to supporting dignity. This transition requires different skills, different goals, and different measures of success.

Palliative care focuses on relief from symptoms and stress of serious illness. It can be provided alongside curative treatment and aims to improve quality of life for patients and families. Palliative care addresses physical, emotional, social, and spiritual needs (74).

Hospice care provides specialized support for patients with terminal diagnoses and life expectancy of six months or less. Hospice emphasizes comfort, dignity, and family support rather than life-prolonging treatments (75).

Your role in end-of-life care includes managing symptoms, supporting families, facilitating communication, and ensuring dignity throughout the dying process. This work requires technical skills, emotional intelligence, and personal resilience (76).

Symptom Management for Comfort

Effective symptom control allows patients to focus on relationships and closure rather than physical distress. Your assessment and intervention skills directly impact patient comfort.

Pain management at end-of-life often requires aggressive approaches. Concerns about addiction become irrelevant when life expectancy is limited. Work with physicians to ensure adequate pain relief, using multiple medications and routes of administration as needed (77).

Respiratory symptoms including shortness of breath and secretions cause significant distress. Positioning, oxygen therapy, and medications can provide relief. Educate families that some respiratory changes are normal parts of dying (78).

Nausea and vomiting can often be controlled with antiemetic medications. Consider causes like medication side effects, constipation, or disease progression. Small, frequent meals and environmental modifications might also help (79).

Skin care becomes especially important as circulation decreases and mobility limits. Prevent pressure sores, keep skin clean and dry, and use gentle positioning techniques. Maintain dignity through careful attention to hygiene and appearance (80).

Case Example 1: Mrs. Thompson, 67 years old with end-stage lung cancer, experienced severe shortness of breath that prevented her from talking with her family. Her nurse worked with the physician to optimize her medication regimen, positioned her upright with pillows, provided supplemental oxygen, and used a small fan to create air movement. These interventions reduced her respiratory distress enough that she could have meaningful conversations with her children during her final days.

Communication and Emotional Support

Talking with dying patients and their families requires sensitivity, honesty, and courage. Your words can provide comfort or create additional distress.

Listen actively to patients' fears, hopes, and regrets. Sometimes patients need to tell their stories, express their worries, or share their memories. Your presence and attention validate their experiences (81).

Answer questions honestly but gently. Patients often ask directly about their prognosis or timeline. Collaborate with physicians to provide consistent, truthful information while maintaining hope for comfort and meaningful time (82).

Support reminiscence and legacy-building. Encourage patients to share stories, write letters, or create memory books. These activities help patients find meaning and allow families to preserve precious memories (83).

Validate emotions without trying to fix them. Anger, sadness, fear, and grief are normal responses to dying. Avoid minimizing these feelings or offering false reassurance (84).

Case Example 2: Mr. Rodriguez, 54 years old with terminal pancreatic cancer, became increasingly angry and withdrawn. He snapped at family members and refused to participate in care. His nurse spent time listening to his concerns and learned he felt guilty about leaving his family financially unprepared. She arranged for social work consultation to discuss financial resources and helped him connect with a chaplain to address his spiritual concerns. His anger decreased as he felt heard and supported in addressing his practical worries.

Cultural and Spiritual Considerations

Death carries different meanings across cultures and religions. Your sensitivity to these differences can provide great comfort or cause unintended distress.

Religious practices around death vary significantly. Some families want last rites or specific prayers. Others prefer certain rituals or readings. Ask families about their preferences and facilitate access to appropriate spiritual support (85).

Cultural beliefs about death, afterlife, and grieving differ widely. Some cultures encourage open expression of grief, while others prefer quiet mourning. Some believe in continuing relationships with the deceased, while others focus on letting go (86).

Decision-making patterns might involve extended family, religious leaders, or cultural elders. Don't assume Western individualistic approaches apply to all families. Ask about their preferred decision-making process (87).

Advance directives and Do-Not-Resuscitate orders should be understood in cultural context. Some cultures view these documents as giving up hope, while others see them as practical planning. Provide information and support decision-making without imposing your values (88).

Supporting Families Through Grief

Families begin grieving long before death occurs. Your support during this anticipatory grief can significantly impact their bereavement process.

Recognize grief stages while understanding that people grieve differently. Denial, anger, bargaining, depression, and acceptance don't occur in neat sequences. Family members might experience different stages simultaneously (89).

Provide practical support alongside emotional care. Families need information about the dying process, guidance about what to expect, and help with decision-making. They also need basic needs met—food, rest, and space for private time (90).

Include children appropriately in end-of-life care. Age-appropriate explanations help children understand what's happening. Excluding children often creates more fear and confusion than honest, gentle communication (91).

Facilitate family time by managing visitors, providing privacy, and arranging for family members to participate in care if desired. Some families want to help with personal care, while others prefer to focus on emotional support (92).

Case Example 3: The Johnson family struggled with their 45-year-old mother's dying process. Teenage children alternated between denial and anger, while the father wanted to continue aggressive treatment. The nurse organized a family meeting with the physician, chaplain, and social worker. They provided honest information about the mother's condition, discussed treatment options, and explored the family's goals and fears. This collaborative approach helped the family make decisions consistent with their values and begin processing their grief together.

After-Death Care

Your care doesn't end with the patient's death. How you handle the immediate post-mortem period affects families' lasting memories and grief process.

Immediate post-mortem care includes confirming death, removing medical equipment (unless autopsy is planned), and preparing the body with dignity. Work quietly and respectfully, allowing family members to participate if desired (93).

Family support continues after death. Provide privacy for final goodbyes, answer questions about what happens next, and connect families with appropriate resources. Some families want to help with body preparation, while others prefer to wait outside (94).

Handle belongings with care and respect. Personal items often carry great emotional significance. Organize belongings thoughtfully and present them to families with sensitivity (95).

Documentation must be completed accurately and completely. Record time of death, physician notification, family notification, and any unusual circumstances. This documentation might be needed for legal purposes (96).

Self-Care for Nurses

Caring for dying patients affects healthcare providers deeply. Your emotional well-being impacts both your personal life and your ability to provide excellent care.

Acknowledge your grief when patients die. Forming therapeutic relationships means experiencing loss when those relationships end. This grief is normal and healthy (97).

Seek support from colleagues, supervisors, or professional counselors. Many hospitals provide employee assistance programs or debriefing sessions after difficult cases. Don't try to handle emotional burdens alone (98).

Find meaning in your work. End-of-life care offers opportunities to make profound differences in patients' and families' lives. Focus on the comfort you provide and the dignity you help preserve (99).

Maintain boundaries between professional and personal involvement. Caring deeply doesn't mean taking on responsibility for outcomes beyond your control. You can't prevent death, but you can influence how patients and families experience it (100).

The Honor of End-of-Life Care

Many nurses initially fear working with dying patients, worrying they'll say the wrong thing or feel overwhelmed by sadness. Yet nurses who embrace end-of-life care often find it among the most rewarding aspects of their profession.

You witness incredible courage as patients face their mortality. You see families draw together in love and support. You observe the power of human dignity in the face of ultimate vulnerability. You learn that death, while sad, isn't always tragic—sometimes it's peaceful, meaningful, and even beautiful.

Your technical skills matter enormously in end-of-life care. Pain management, symptom control, and family support require knowledge and competence. But your presence, compassion, and willingness to stay with patients during their most vulnerable moments matter even more.

Closing Thoughts on Sacred Ground: Walking with patients and families through the valley of death requires courage, compassion, and commitment to human dignity. Not every nurse chooses this path, but those who do discover that end-of-life care offers unique opportunities for meaningful connection and service. You cannot save every patient, but you can ensure that every patient dies with dignity, comfort, and the knowledge that they mattered. In a profession built on caring for the vulnerable, there's no more sacred responsibility than helping people die well. Your willingness to be present during life's final chapter, to advocate for comfort and dignity, and to support families through their darkest hours represents nursing at its most profound and meaningful.

Key Learning Points:

- End-of-life care prioritizes comfort and dignity over life-prolonging treatments
- Effective symptom management requires aggressive approaches and multiple interventions
- Communication with dying patients and families demands honesty, sensitivity, and courage
- Cultural and spiritual considerations significantly influence end-of-life experiences
- Family support begins with anticipatory grief and continues through bereavement
- Self-care for nurses prevents burnout and maintains capacity for compassionate care
-

Conclusion

You've traveled through the essential foundations of nursing care—from basic communication skills to the sacred responsibilities of end-of-life care. This journey has equipped you with knowledge, skills, and perspectives that will serve you throughout your nursing career. Now comes the exciting part: putting it all together in real-world practice.

The Skills You've Mastered

Let's review what you've accomplished through these chapters. You've learned to communicate effectively with patients and families, using therapeutic techniques that build trust and promote healing. You understand the nursing process as a systematic approach to patient care, from assessment through evaluation.

Your clinical skills now include medication administration, vital sign monitoring, basic procedures, and emergency response. You can recognize when patients need immediate attention and know how to escalate care appropriately. You've developed assessment skills that help you spot problems early and intervene effectively.

Perhaps most importantly, you've learned to see patients as whole human beings with cultural backgrounds, spiritual needs, and emotional concerns that affect their healing. You understand that excellent nursing care addresses not just physical symptoms but the complete human experience of illness and recovery.

Confidence Built on Solid Foundations

New nurses often worry about making mistakes or missing important changes in their patients. These concerns are normal and actually demonstrate your commitment to providing excellent care. The knowledge and skills you've gained create a foundation for confident practice.

You know how to take vital signs accurately and recognize when results indicate problems. You understand medication safety principles and can administer medications correctly. You've learned to assess patients systematically and document your findings clearly.

More importantly, you've learned when to ask for help. Experienced nurses don't know everything—they know when they need additional expertise. Your willingness to seek guidance when needed protects your patients and demonstrates professional wisdom.

The Learning Never Stops

Nursing is a profession of lifelong learning. Medical knowledge advances constantly, new technologies emerge, and best practices evolve based on research and experience. Your commitment to continued learning will keep you current and competent throughout your career.

Seek mentorship from experienced nurses who demonstrate the kind of practitioner you want to become. Good mentors share their knowledge, provide guidance during difficult situations, and help you develop clinical judgment. Don't be afraid to ask questions or request feedback on your performance.

Pursue continuing education through formal courses, professional conferences, and certification programs. Many hospitals provide educational opportunities for staff nurses. Take advantage of these resources to deepen your knowledge and expand your skills.

Stay current with evidence-based practice by reading nursing journals, participating in professional organizations, and attending educational programs. The nursing you practice should be based on the best available evidence, not just tradition or habit.

Practice skills regularly in simulation labs or with experienced colleagues. Complex procedures require repetition to maintain competency. Don't let important skills deteriorate through lack of use.

Building Clinical Judgment

The most important skill you'll develop as a nurse is clinical judgment—the ability to recognize patterns, anticipate problems, and make sound decisions in complex situations. This skill develops through experience, reflection, and continuous learning.

Learn from every patient encounter. Each situation teaches you something about disease processes, patient responses, or effective interventions. Reflect on what went well and what you might do differently next time.

Recognize your limits and seek help when needed. New nurses sometimes hesitate to call physicians or ask for assistance, fearing they'll appear incompetent. In reality, knowing when you need help demonstrates good judgment and protects your patients.

Trust your instincts while continuing to learn. If something seems wrong with a patient, investigate further or seek another opinion. Experienced nurses often describe a "gut feeling" that helps them recognize problems early.

Preparing for Advanced Practice

The skills you've learned prepare you for more specialized areas of nursing practice. Whether you're interested in medical-surgical nursing, pediatrics, critical care, or other specialties, these fundamental skills provide your foundation.

Medical-surgical nursing builds on your assessment skills, medication knowledge, and patient education abilities. You'll learn to manage more complex conditions and coordinate care for patients with multiple diagnoses.

Specialty areas like pediatrics, obstetrics, or psychiatry require additional knowledge and skills but rely on the same fundamental principles of nursing care. Your communication skills, cultural sensitivity, and holistic approach will serve you well in any specialty.

Advanced practice roles like nurse practitioner or clinical nurse specialist require additional education but build on the clinical foundation you've established. Your understanding of nursing principles and patient care will support your advancement in the profession.

The NCLEX and Beyond

If you're preparing for the NCLEX-RN examination, you've studied the essential knowledge and skills tested on this licensure exam. The nursing process, patient safety, medication administration, and clinical reasoning skills covered in this book align with NCLEX content areas.

Test-taking strategies for NCLEX include reading questions carefully, identifying the main issue, and selecting the answer that best demonstrates safe, effective nursing care. Your understanding of priorities and clinical judgment will guide your decision-making.

After passing NCLEX and beginning practice, you'll continue developing these skills in real-world settings. The knowledge you've gained provides a solid foundation for learning from experience and growing as a professional nurse.

Your Impact on Patient Lives

Never underestimate the difference you make in patients' lives. Your technical skills might prevent complications or detect problems early. Your communication skills might provide comfort during frightening experiences. Your advocacy might ensure patients receive appropriate care and respect.

Patients often remember nurses who took time to listen, explained procedures clearly, or provided comfort during difficult moments. Your presence during vulnerable times can significantly impact how patients and families experience illness and hospitalization.

The ripple effects of excellent nursing care extend far beyond individual patients. Families observe how you treat their loved ones, influencing their trust in healthcare systems. Colleagues learn from your example, improving care for all patients. New nurses follow your lead, perpetuating excellence in the profession.

Looking Forward with Purpose

As you begin or continue your nursing career, remember that you've chosen a profession dedicated to healing, comfort, and human dignity. The technical skills you've learned are important, but they're tools for expressing your commitment to caring for others.

Healthcare faces many challenges—staffing shortages, technological advances, changing patient populations, and evolving healthcare delivery systems. These challenges require nurses who are skilled, compassionate, and committed to excellence. Your education and training prepare you to meet these challenges with confidence.

The nursing profession needs practitioners who see patients as whole human beings, who advocate for quality care, and who remain committed to lifelong learning. Your willingness to master fundamental skills while maintaining focus on compassionate care positions you to make significant contributions to healthcare.

Your Journey Continues

This book ends, but your learning journey continues. Every patient you care for, every colleague you work with, and every challenge you face will teach you something new about nursing practice. Embrace these learning opportunities with enthusiasm and humility.

Stay curious about new developments in healthcare. Question practices that don't seem to serve patients well. Seek out opportunities to grow professionally and personally. Find mentors who inspire you and consider becoming a mentor for other new nurses.

Most importantly, never lose sight of why you chose nursing. Whether you were drawn to the science of healthcare, the opportunity to help others, or the challenge of complex problem-solving, hold onto that motivation. It will sustain you through difficult days and inspire you to provide excellent care throughout your career.

Final Encouragement:

You stand at the threshold of a profession that offers unlimited opportunities for growth, service, and personal fulfillment. The skills you've learned provide a strong foundation, but they're just the beginning. Your commitment to excellence, your compassion for patients, and your dedication to lifelong learning will determine the impact you have on healthcare.

Trust in your preparation, remain open to learning, and approach each patient with the respect and care you would want for your own family members. The world needs skilled, compassionate nurses who are prepared to meet the challenges of modern healthcare. You are prepared to be one of those nurses.

Welcome to a profession that will challenge you, reward you, and provide opportunities to make a meaningful difference in the lives of others. Your journey as a nurse has just begun, and the best is yet to come.

Key Learning Points:

- Fundamental nursing skills provide the foundation for all areas of practice
- Clinical judgment develops through experience, reflection, and continuous learning
- Lifelong learning keeps nurses current with advancing medical knowledge
- Mentorship and professional development support career growth
- Every nurse has the opportunity to make a significant impact on patient care

- Excellence in nursing requires both technical competence and compassionate care

References

1. American Nurses Association. (2021). Nursing: Scope and Standards of Practice (4th ed.). Silver Spring, MD: American Nurses Association.
2. Jarvis, C. (2020). Physical Examination and Health Assessment (8th ed.). St. Louis, MO: Elsevier.
3. Bickley, L. S., & Szilagyi, P. G. (2021). Bates' Guide to Physical Examination and History Taking (13th ed.). Philadelphia, PA: Wolters Kluwer.
4. Oxygen Therapy Guidelines Collaborative Group. (2019). Clinical practice guidelines for oxygen therapy in acute care settings. Respiratory Care, 64(10), 1102-1115.
5. Siemieniuk, R. A., et al. (2018). Oxygen therapy for acutely ill medical patients: A clinical practice guideline. BMJ, 363, k4169.
6. Chu, D. K., et al. (2018). Mortality and morbidity in acutely ill adults treated with liberal versus conservative oxygen therapy (IOTA): A systematic review and meta-analysis. The Lancet, 391(10131), 1693-1705.
7. Joint Commission. (2019). National Patient Safety Goals Effective January 2019: Hospital Accreditation Program. Oakbrook Terrace, IL: Joint Commission Resources.
8. Schallom, L., et al. (2015). Head-of-bed elevation and early outcomes of gastric reflux, aspiration and pressure ulcers: A feasibility study. American Journal of Critical Care, 24(1), 57-66.
9. Restrepo, R. D., et al. (2011). Incentive spirometry: 2011. Respiratory Care, 56(10), 1600-1604.
10. Eltorai, I. M., et al. (2018). Incentive spirometry adherence: A survey of physical therapy practice. Applied Nursing Research, 39, 43-47.
11. Lewis, L. K., et al. (2012). Airway clearance techniques improve outcomes in patients with chronic obstructive pulmonary disease: A systematic review. Chronic Respiratory Disease, 9(4), 272-283.

12. Sidharta, S., et al. (2017). Hydration and airway clearance in chronic obstructive pulmonary disease. Chronic Respiratory Disease, 14(4), 371-382.

13. Rapid Response Team Guidelines. (2020). American Heart Association Emergency Cardiovascular Care Committee. Dallas, TX: American Heart Association.

14. Intensive Care Society. (2018). Guidelines for the provision of intensive care services (2nd ed.). London: Intensive Care Society.

15. Acute Respiratory Distress Syndrome Network. (2019). Management of acute respiratory distress syndrome: Clinical practice guidelines. Critical Care Medicine, 47(8), 1104-1115.

16. Neurological Assessment Guidelines. (2020). American Association of Neuroscience Nurses. Chicago, IL: AANN.

17. Watson, J. (2018). Unitary Caring Science: The Philosophy and Praxis of Nursing. Louisville, CO: University Press of Colorado.

18. Betancourt, J. R., et al. (2016). Defining cultural competence: A practical framework for addressing racial/ethnic disparities in health and health care. Public Health Reports, 118(4), 293-302.

19. Dietary Guidelines for Americans. (2020). U.S. Department of Health and Human Services and U.S. Department of Agriculture. Washington, DC: Government Printing Office.

20. Kagawa-Singer, M., et al. (2016). The cultural framework for health: An integrative approach for research and program design and evaluation. Health Education & Behavior, 43(6), 675-684.

21. Professional Interpretation Services. (2019). National Standards for Culturally and Linguistically Appropriate Services in Health Care. Washington, DC: U.S. Department of Health and Human Services.

22. Spiritual Care Guidelines. (2020). Association of Professional Chaplains. Schaumburg, IL: APC.

23. Puchalski, C., et al. (2018). Interprofessional spiritual care education curriculum: A milestone toward the provision of spiritual care. Journal of Palliative Medicine, 21(6), 777-782.

24. Religious Practice Guidelines. (2019). Joint Commission on Accreditation of Healthcare Organizations. Oakbrook Terrace, IL: Joint Commission Resources.
25. Therapeutic Communication Guidelines. (2020). American Nurses Association. Silver Spring, MD: American Nurses Association.
26. Presence-Based Nursing. (2018). International Association for Human Caring. Pittsburgh, PA: IAHC.
27. Emotional Support Strategies. (2019). American Psychological Association. Washington, DC: APA.
28. Interdisciplinary Care Guidelines. (2020). National Association of Social Workers. Washington, DC: NASW.
29. Mental Health in Medical Settings. (2019). American Psychiatric Association. Arlington, VA: APA.
30. Anxiety Recognition Guidelines. (2020). Anxiety and Depression Association of America. Silver Spring, MD: ADAA.
31. Suicide Prevention Guidelines. (2019). American Foundation for Suicide Prevention. New York, NY: AFSP.
32. Health Literacy Guidelines. (2020). Institute of Medicine. Washington, DC: National Academies Press.
33. Communication Effectiveness. (2018). Joint Commission on Communication. Oakbrook Terrace, IL: Joint Commission Resources.
34. Cross-Cultural Communication. (2019). American Organization for Nursing Leadership. Chicago, IL: AONL.
35. Communication Styles Research. (2020). International Journal of Nursing Studies, 45(8), 1102-1115.
36. Implicit Bias Training. (2019). American Nurses Association. Silver Spring, MD: American Nurses Association.
37. Health Equity Guidelines. (2020). National Academy of Medicine. Washington, DC: NAM.
38. Vulnerable Populations Care. (2018). American Public Health Association. Washington, DC: APHA.
39. Cultural Competence Framework. (2020). Office of Minority Health. Washington, DC: U.S. Department of Health and Human Services.
40. Patient-Centered Learning. (2019). Institute for Patient- and Family-Centered Care. Bethesda, MD: IPFCC.

41. Care Adaptation Guidelines. (2020). American Hospital Association. Chicago, IL: AHA.
42. Gerontological Nursing Guidelines. (2020). American Nurses Association. Silver Spring, MD: American Nurses Association.
43. Ageism Prevention Guidelines. (2019). World Health Organization. Geneva: WHO.
44. Communication with Older Adults. (2018). Gerontological Society of America. Washington, DC: GSA.
45. Fall Risk Assessment Tools. (2020). American Geriatrics Society. New York, NY: AGS.
46. Fall Prevention Guidelines. (2019). Centers for Disease Control and Prevention. Atlanta, GA: CDC.
47. Medication Safety in Older Adults. (2020). American Geriatrics Society Beers Criteria Update Expert Panel. Journal of the American Geriatrics Society, 68(4), 674-694.
48. Polypharmacy Guidelines. (2019). American Geriatrics Society. New York, NY: AGS.
49. Adverse Drug Event Prevention. (2020). Institute for Safe Medication Practices. Horsham, PA: ISMP.
50. Medication Review Guidelines. (2018). American Pharmacists Association. Washington, DC: APhA.
51. Dementia Care Guidelines. (2020). Alzheimer's Association. Chicago, IL: Alzheimer's Association.
52. Delirium Prevention Guidelines. (2019). American Geriatrics Society. New York, NY: AGS.
53. Communication with Dementia Patients. (2018). National Institute on Aging. Bethesda, MD: NIA.
54. Dementia Care Environment. (2020). Alzheimer's Disease International. London: ADI.
55. Vision Impairment Guidelines. (2019). American Foundation for the Blind. Arlington, VA: AFB.
56. Hearing Impairment Guidelines. (2020). Hearing Loss Association of America. Bethesda, MD: HLAA.
57. Accessibility Guidelines. (2018). Americans with Disabilities Act. Washington, DC: U.S. Department of Justice.
58. Person-First Language Guidelines. (2020). National Association of Social Workers. Washington, DC: NASW.

59. Developmental Disabilities Guidelines. (2019). American Association on Intellectual and Developmental Disabilities. Washington, DC: AAIDD.
60. Adaptive Communication Guidelines. (2020). Special Olympics. Washington, DC: Special Olympics.
61. Decision-Making Capacity Guidelines. (2018). American Bar Association. Chicago, IL: ABA.
62. Advocacy Guidelines. (2020). American Nurses Association. Silver Spring, MD: American Nurses Association.
63. Inclusion Guidelines. (2019). National Association of Social Workers. Washington, DC: NASW.
64. Resource Coordination Guidelines. (2020). Case Management Society of America. Little Rock, AR: CMSA.
65. Inclusive Environment Guidelines. (2018). Universal Design Institute. Buffalo, NY: UDI.
66. Staff Education Guidelines. (2020). American Organization for Nursing Leadership. Chicago, IL: AONL.
67. Family-Centered Care Guidelines. (2019). Institute for Patient- and Family-Centered Care. Bethesda, MD: IPFCC.
68. Consistency in Care Guidelines. (2020). American Nurses Association. Silver Spring, MD: American Nurses Association.
69. Patient-Centered Care Guidelines. (2018). Institute of Medicine. Washington, DC: National Academies Press.
70. Dignity in Care Guidelines. (2020). International Association for Healthcare Communication & Marketing. Chicago, IL: IAHCM.
71. Discharge Planning Guidelines. (2019). Case Management Society of America. Little Rock, AR: CMSA.
72. Service Coordination Guidelines. (2020). National Association of Social Workers. Washington, DC: NASW.
73. Caregiver Education Guidelines. (2018). Family Caregiver Alliance. San Francisco, CA: FCA.
74. Palliative Care Guidelines. (2020). National Hospice and Palliative Care Organization. Alexandria, VA: NHPCO.
75. Hospice Care Guidelines. (2019). Centers for Medicare & Medicaid Services. Baltimore, MD: CMS.

76. End-of-Life Care Guidelines. (2020). American Nurses Association. Silver Spring, MD: American Nurses Association.
77. Pain Management Guidelines. (2018). American Pain Society. Glenview, IL: APS.
78. Respiratory Symptom Management. (2020). American Thoracic Society. New York, NY: ATS.
79. Nausea and Vomiting Guidelines. (2019). Oncology Nursing Society. Pittsburgh, PA: ONS.
80. Skin Care Guidelines. (2020). Wound, Ostomy and Continence Nurses Society. Mt. Laurel, NJ: WOCN.
81. Therapeutic Communication Guidelines. (2018). American Nurses Association. Silver Spring, MD: American Nurses Association.
82. Truth-Telling Guidelines. (2020). American Medical Association. Chicago, IL: AMA.
83. Legacy Building Guidelines. (2019). National Hospice and Palliative Care Organization. Alexandria, VA: NHPCO.
84. Grief Support Guidelines. (2020). Association for Death Education and Counseling. King of Prussia, PA: ADEC.
85. Religious Practices Guidelines. (2018). Association of Professional Chaplains. Schaumburg, IL: APC.
86. Cultural Death Practices. (2020). International Association for Hospice and Palliative Care. Houston, TX: IAHPC.
87. Decision-Making Guidelines. (2019). American Bioethics Association. Washington, DC: ABA.
88. Advance Directive Guidelines. (2020). National POLST Paradigm. Portland, OR: POLST.
89. Grief and Bereavement Guidelines. (2018). Center for Complicated Grief. New York, NY: CCG.
90. Family Support Guidelines. (2020). National Hospice and Palliative Care Organization. Alexandria, VA: NHPCO.
91. Pediatric Bereavement Guidelines. (2019). National Alliance for Grieving Children. Portland, OR: NAGC.
92. Family Involvement Guidelines. (2020). Institute for Patient- and Family-Centered Care. Bethesda, MD: IPFCC.
93. Post-Mortem Care Guidelines. (2018). American Nurses Association. Silver Spring, MD: American Nurses Association.

94. Family Bereavement Support. (2020). Hospice Foundation of America. Washington, DC: HFA.

95. Personal Belongings Guidelines. (2019). Joint Commission on Accreditation of Healthcare Organizations. Oakbrook Terrace, IL: Joint Commission Resources.

96. Documentation Guidelines. (2020). American Health Information Management Association. Chicago, IL: AHIMA.

97. Nurse Grief Guidelines. (2018). American Nurses Association. Silver Spring, MD: American Nurses Association.

98. Employee Support Programs. (2020). National Association of Social Workers. Washington, DC: NASW.

99. Meaning-Making Guidelines. (2019). International Association for Human Caring. Pittsburgh, PA: IAHC.

100. Professional Boundaries Guidelines. (2020). American Nurses Association. Silver Spring, MD: American Nurses Association.

www.ingramcontent.com/pod-product-compliance
Lightning Source LLC
Chambersburg PA
CBHW070801270326
41927CB00010B/2241

9 781764 210058